THE PLANTAR FASCIITIS BIBLE

By Benn J S Boshell

Published by Benn Boshell

First published 2017

© Benn Boshell

The moral right of the author has been asserted.

All rights reserved. Without limiting the rights under copyright restricted above, no part of this publication may be reproduced, stored in or introduced into a retrieval system, or transmitted in any form or by any means (electronic, mechanical, photocopying, recording or otherwise), without the prior written permission of the copyright owner and the above publisher of this book.

About the Author

Benn J S Boshell is a Podiatrist with a specialist interest in heel pain. He set up the YouTube channel in 2012 *'Plantar Fasciitis Gone'* which is a free patient education resource that has helped thousands of plantar fasciitis sufferers all over the world. Benn graduated from the University of Southampton in 2010 with a BSc (Hons) degree in Podiatry. Benn has also completed an MSc degree in Podiatric Surgery at The University of Brighton which has allowed him to further improve his knowledge and clinical practice. Benn currently works in full-time private practice in Wiltshire & Somerset, UK.

Disclaimer

This book is not intended to substitute any kind of medical advice. Readers of this book should seek professional medical advice from a foot specialist prior to following any recommendations made by the author.

Table of Contents

Chapter One: Introduction 7
    Mission Statement 7
    There Are No Secrets 8
    The First Port of Call - The GP 9

Chapter Two: Plantar Fascia Anatomy 11
    Central Band of Plantar Fascia 11
    Medial Band of Plantar Fascia 12
    Lateral Band of Plantar Fascia 12

Chapter Three: Plantar Fasciitis FAQs 14
    What is Plantar Fasciitis? (fashee-EYE-tiss) 14
    What causes it? 15
    What are the symptoms of plantar fasciitis? 15
    How is plantar fasciitis diagnosed? 16
    Why did I get plantar fasciitis? 16
    Is it treatable? 17
    How long will it take for the pain to go away? 17
    What causes treatment to fail? 18
    How do I prevent the pain recurring? 18

Chapter Four: Treatment Options 20
    Relative Rest 21
    Stretching Exercises 22
    Night Splints 25
    Orthoses (Insoles) 29
    Footwear Modification 33
    Extra-corporeal Shockwave Therapy (ESWT) 35
    Weight Loss 37
    Taping 42
    Corticosteroid Injections 43
    Therapeutic Ultrasound 45
    Immobilisation 48

Botulinum Toxin A (Botox) Injections 50
Trigger Point Therapy 54
Surgery 57

Chapter Five: Heel Pain Differential Diagnoses: Other Causes of Heel Pain 59

Heel Pain of Neural Origin 59
Inflammatory Disease and Heel Pain 65
Sarcoidosis and Heel Pain 72
Heel pain and Hyperparathyroidism 73
Heel pain and Sickle Cell Anaemia 74
Plantar Fibromatosis 75
Plantar Fascia Rupture 77

Chapter Six: Diagnostic Modalities for Heel Pain 79

X-rays 79
Diagnostic Ultrasound 80
MRI 81
Computerized Tomography (CT) Scan 81
Technetium 99 Bone Scan 81
Electrodiagnostic study 82
Pressure-specific sensory testing 83

Chapter Seven: Soft Tissue Stress & Injury to the Plantar Fascia 84

Physiological Stress (normal injury free stress) 84

Chapter Eight: Biomechanical Theory of Plantar Fasciitis 87

The Windlass Mechanism 88

Chapter Nine: Miscellaneous Topics 90

Plantar Fasciitis or Heel Spur? 90
Tight Hamstrings Linked to Plantar Fasciitis 95
Plantar Fascia Friendly Exercise 97
Prefabricated orthoses or custom made orthoses? 99
Wearing a Night Splint 100
More on Trigger Point Therapy 102
Leg Length Discrepancy and Plantar Fasciitis 105

Chapter Ten: Final Thoughts 109

Bibliography 112

Chapter One

Introduction

Mission Statement

Firstly, thank you for purchasing this book. During my training as a podiatrist, it occurred to me just how common plantar fasciitis is. It affects a whopping 10% of the general population. It then became apparent to me how poor most patient's understanding is of this common condition partly due to the misinformation they had been provided with about plantar fasciitis. What's worse, is that this misinformation sometimes came from qualified health professionals. It became very apparent that most patients and some qualified professionals generally have a poor understanding of plantar fasciitis and how to manage it. This is probably not helped by the difficult pronunciation of the word fasciitis (fashee-eye-tiss). Patient education is at the heart of successful healthcare. The greater the understanding a patient has about their medical condition the more likely they are to successfully manage their condition. This education also relies on accurate information being provided to patients from health professionals. Hence the aim of this E-book is to educate patients, healthcare students, and qualified professionals about plantar fasciitis. This E-book provides impartial **evidence-based** information that is reader friendly so patients can understand their condition and make well-informed decisions on how to manage it.

https://www.youtube.com/user/PlantarFasciitisGone

There Are No Secrets

After setting up my YouTube channel Plantar Fasciitis Gone (https://www.youtube.com/user/PlantarFasciitsGone) in 2012 I noticed that there are a wide number of online resources to help patients with plantar fasciitis ranging from other YouTube videos, blogs, independent websites set up by plantar fasciitis sufferers who share their stories and what has helped them with their pain etc. There is also a large number of books, E-books, and DVDs claiming to hold *"secrets"* on how to cure plantar fasciitis.

Time for a reality check. Here is the bitter truth. There are no secrets to cure plantar fasciitis. There is no magical exercise, supplement, medicine, guru, genie or wizard who can guarantee to cure plantar fasciitis as some of them claim. It is a ridiculous claim that any treatment can guarantee to cure a musculoskeletal problem such as plantar fasciitis, in the same way, that there are no secrets to cure other very common musculoskeletal injuries such as shin splints, ITB syndrome, patellofemoral pain syndrome, tennis elbow, Achilles tendinitis etc. Though some will have you believe it. Unfortunately for some patients who continue to suffer from plantar fasciitis despite having tried nearly all of the available treatment options they start to become desperate for a cure which in turn can make them gullible enough to believe that there are secrets or quick fixes that the medical profession isn't letting them know about. No one ethical can guarantee you that they can cure your plantar fasciitis and nor do I. I hope reading this page alone with save you thousands in money.

Ok, rant over.

The First Port of Call - The GP

When a patient suffers from foot pain their first port of call is often to visit their General Practitioner (GP). Most UK GP's will confirm that they see a high number of foot complaints which they diagnose as plantar fasciitis. For some GP's diagnosing plantar fasciitis is simple enough after taking a patient history and conducting a physical examination but what comes next is more challenging. How to cure it? There is a lack of consistent advice given to patients on how to manage plantar fasciitis with some telling the patient *"to do nothing, it is a self-resolving condition and that it will go away by itself after 2 years."* Whilst others tell their patients they have *"flat feet"* and tell them to go and buy some insoles. Also, it is not uncommon for GP's to even provide a corticosteroid injection as a first line therapy for plantar fasciitis and then send the patient on their way with the hope that this will be a long-term solution to the problem. Furthermore, a commonly reported scenario from patients is that they went to their GP who referred them for an x-ray and was then diagnosed as having a heel spur based on the x-ray result and advised that nothing can be done unless they have it surgically removed. This kind of advice is erroneous.

So is your GP to blame for poor care?

Not exactly. It is well known that musculoskeletal medicine is not a priority subject for medical students during their training, nor is it a priority for newly qualified doctors unless they express a specialist interest in this field or progress their training in this subject area. They have a lot to study about the human body and unfortunately, musculoskeletal medicine takes a back seat for more life-threatening conditions such as cardiovascular disease, respiratory disease, infectious diseases, cancer etc. Generally, this results in a limited knowledge base on musculoskeletal conditions. So if the patients first port of call is often the GP it is obvious how they can start their treatment on the wrong foot (excuse the pun).

So what should your GP do?

If your GP is well informed on foot pain and can competently make a diagnosis of plantar fasciitis and then advise you on evidence-based treatment options that will provide a realistic long term solution to your plantar fasciitis then that is the most one can ask for. If your GP doesn't possess this knowledge then they should refer you to a suitably qualified professional, usually a podiatrist or a physiotherapist.

Chapter Two

Plantar Fascia Anatomy

In order for patients and professionals to understand plantar fasciitis, they must have at least a simple appreciation of the anatomy of the plantar fascia. In short, the plantar fascia has 3 main portions:

1. central band
2. medial band
3. lateral band

The reason you need to know this is because together the plantar fascia covers a large area of the foot and not everybody experiences plantar fasciitis in the same place or indeed in the same band.

Central Band of Plantar Fascia

The central band is by far the most common injury site in plantar fasciitis and usually, occurs at its attachment to the medial calcaneal tuberosity (the bottom of the heel bone). Pain can also be experienced approximately 2-5cm beyond the heel bone into the sole of the foot with tenderness running along to the ends of the toes.

Medial Band of Plantar Fascia

The medial band is thin and forms the covering of the abductor hallucis muscle (muscle along the inside of the arch). It can also become painful in plantar fasciitis. Pain along the medial band is experienced more along the side of the heel bone and along the inside of the arch.

Lateral Band of Plantar Fascia

The least common type of plantar fasciitis is pain along the lateral band which is a much smaller, less significant portion of the plantar fascia by comparison to the other two bands. It is also attached to medial calcaneal tubercle like the central band is, however, is continues along the outer side of the heel to attach to the base of the 5th metatarsal. Pain in the lateral band is experienced more towards the outer part of the heel.

Why you need to know this

The location of your pain will be dependent on what part of the plantar fascia you have injured. For example, if you have injured the medial band of the plantar fascia you may experience pain on the inside of the heel or along the inside of the arch in the foot. This area of pain does not fit the classic description of "plantar fasciitis" which is in most cases painful at the bottom of the heel. Therefore when patients self-diagnose their foot pain thanks to all the wonderful and sometimes shambolic information available via the internet they may end up believing they have a different condition because the information they have read doesn't fit their profile.

<u>Advice - Do not self-diagnose your pain. This can result in inappropriate treatment, a risk of harm and delayed recovery.</u>

Seek professional advice from a podiatrist or suitably qualified health professional. The first step to successful treatment is the correct diagnosis

Chapter Three

Plantar Fasciitis FAQs

What is Plantar Fasciitis? (fashee-EYE-tiss)

Plantar fasciitis is a common painful foot condition located mostly at the heel. Although originally thought of as an inflammatory process, plantar fasciitis is a disorder of degenerative changes in the plantar fascia leading to thickening of the fibre and may be more accurately termed plantar fasciosis (Lemont et al 2003). Plantar means the bottom of the foot, and fascia is the fibrous tissues that connect the heel bone (calcaneus) to the heads of the metatarsal bones found at the base of your toes. It is an overuse injury where the plantar fascia becomes strained due to levels of stress that exceed how much the plantar fascia can tolerate. The level of stress the plantar fascia can tolerate varies from person to person. Plantar fasciitis is the most common cause of heel pain affecting up to 10% of the population. It is most often seen in middle-aged men and women (between the ages 40-60), but can be found in all age groups and is also common in the athletic population (Rome et al 2001). In these athletes, it is thought that the repetitive nature of the sports causes the damage to the plantar fascia.

What causes it?

The cause of plantar fasciitis is multi-factorial meaning that it is caused by a combination of individual factors. There is no one single cause of the condition. Proposed causative factors in the medical literature can be split into two types:

Intrinsic factors:

- feet that roll inwards too much when walking (increased pronation)
- feet with very low arches (flat feet)
- feet with very high arches
- tight Achilles tendons or calf muscles
- tight hamstrings
- limited ankle joint flexibility
- being overweight

Extrinsic factors:

- Occupations that keep you on your feet. Factory workers, teachers, chefs, nurses, cleaners and others who spend most of their work hours walking or standing on hard surfaces can damage their plantar fascia.
- Improper shoes – shoes that are not supportive or worn out.

What are the symptoms of plantar fasciitis?

Plantar fasciitis is diagnosed clinically with the classic symptoms of "sharp/stabbing" pain well localized over the heel area of the bottom of the foot as this is where the plantar fascia attaches to the heel bone. Often the pain from plantar fasciitis is most severe when you first stand on your feet in the morning. Pain often subsides after a while, but then returns after prolonged standing or walking.

Typically pain is noticeable when standing after a long period of rest, this is known as post-static dyskinesia.

The pain is often described as a sharp, stabbing pain and can feel like walking on a marble. In some cases, pain may also extend along the sole of the foot where the plantar fascia continues to attach to the metatarsal heads.

How is plantar fasciitis diagnosed?

The diagnosis of plantar fasciitis is usually made by a patient history that matches the classical symptoms of plantar fasciitis, along with a clinical assessment by a podiatrist or suitably qualified health professional. Diagnostic imaging such as ultrasound and MRI are not routinely used to confirm a diagnosis but can be helpful when one is unsure of the diagnosis. Diagnostic imaging is also useful to rule out differential diagnoses such as radiculopathy (referred back pain), bone oedema, plantar fascia tear, fracture, inflammatory disorders etc.

Why did I get plantar fasciitis?

Plantar fasciitis occurs because of irritation to the thick ligamentous connective tissue that runs from the heel bone to the ball of the foot. This strong and tight tissue contributes to maintaining the arch of the foot.

It is also one of the major transmitters of weight across the foot as you walk or run. Therefore, the stress placed on this tissue is tremendous. When the amount of stress placed on the plantar fascia exceeds the amount it can tolerate it becomes damaged causing the connective tissue that forms the arch of the foot to become thickened and degenerative. The reason one may have placed too much stress on their plantar fascia varies greatly from person to person. For some, it may be a combination of tight calf muscles and feet that pronate (roll in). For others, it may be standing for long periods in unsuitable footwear. All of these individual factors contribute to the loading stress on the plantar fascia.

Is it treatable?

Of course, it is! This book would be a lot shorter if there was absolutely no hope. But no single treatment works best for everyone with plantar fasciitis. The most important thing is to identify and eliminate the causative factor(s), which again differs from person to person. Fortunately, there are many things you can try to help your foot get better:

- *A short period of rest – cut back on activities that make the pain worse*
- *Ice treatment to reduce pain*
- *Massage which often provides a therapeutic effect*
- *Wearing a night splint*
- *Following a prescribed stretching and strengthening programme*
- *Wearing appropriate shoes*
- *Wearing functional foot orthoses (insoles)*

This list is not exhaustive. We will cover available treatments in more depth in chapter four.

How long will it take for the pain to go away?

This is a tough question as there are many factors that can influence one's healing such as their overall medical health, certain medical conditions are known to delay one's capacity to heal from injury such as diabetes, immune deficiencies, poor blood supply etc. Plantar fasciitis most often occurs because of repetitive micro-trauma injuries that have happened over time. The length of time you have had the condition also influences how well it will respond to treatment. What we know is that chronic conditions (over 6 months) are more difficult to heal and less respondent to conventional treatment. Therefore the quicker you receive treatment the better chance you have in curing the problem.

What causes treatment to fail?

Nonsurgical treatments almost always improve the pain. It is commonly reported that 90% of cases will get better from nonsurgical treatment. If the underlying causes of plantar fasciitis are properly addressed patients usually respond very well to treatment.

Reasons for treatment failing are most commonly due to inappropriate treatment recommended, and poor patient compliance i.e. not wearing appropriate footwear or not performing prescribed treatments correctly. Treatment may also fail in chronic plantar fasciitis (having the condition for over 6 months). In chronic cases, the plantar fascia may become very degenerative with a build up of scar tissue. This makes the condition more difficult to treat and less responsive to conventional treatment. In chronic cases, one may benefit from treatments aiming to promote and restart the healing cascade such as extra-corporeal shockwave therapy. We will cover this treatment option in more detail later on.

Another cause for treatment to fail is misdiagnosis where the cause of the pain is in fact not plantar fasciitis but instead a different type of heel pain.

How do I prevent the pain recurring?

One of the most important things is to maintain your improved flexibility since muscular tightness is one of the leading causes of plantar fasciitis. This can be achieved by performing stretching exercises once every few days or as often as you start to notice any tightening of your muscles. Maintaining the improved flexibility reduces your chances of going back to square one.

It is equally important to wear appropriate shoes. This does not mean you have to spend all of the time in supportive footwear. It simply means that spending all of your time in bad footwear will increase the likelihood of the condition recurring.

Chapter Four

Treatment Options

Relative Rest

Stretching Exercises

Night Splints

Orthoses (Insoles)

Massage

Footwear modifications

Extra-corporeal Shockwave Therapy

Weight Loss

Strengthening Exercises

Taping

Corticosteroid Injections

Ultrasound

Acupuncture

Immobilisation

Platelet Rich Plasma (PRP) Injections

Botulinum Toxin A (Botox) Injections

Trigger Point Therapy

Radiotherapy

Surgery

As you can see from the list there is a multitude of treatment options available for treating plantar fasciitis, with some more successful than others. In order to make this section as reader friendly as possible the discussed treatment options will be broken down as follows.

Rationale – this explains the reasoning behind the proposed treatment

Evidence – the current research which supports or refutes its effectiveness in the treatment of plantar fasciitis

Risks – the potential risks of the individual treatment modality

Verdict – this is the professional opinion of the author

This chapter is presented in an easy to read, the overview of the current evidence base for plantar fasciitis treatments for patients and professionals and is not an academic, systematic review. It does not provide a full critical analysis on the strength/quality of the referenced research studies but will mention limitations of the research when necessary.

Relative Rest

Rationale

An obvious option to most, but not everyone follows this simple yet vital step. *Relative* rest does not mean any activity or weight bearing at all. What it means is a modification to your current day to day regime so that you are minimising activities which make your pain worse. For some, this may be reducing the weekly mileage or frequency of running if their pain is linked to running or that they suffer the day after a run. For more severe cases it may mean complete rest from running until the pain has improved. If you notice that spending excessively long hours on your feet aggravates your symptoms then try to reduce the amount of time you spend on your feet. This is difficult for people whose job role requires periods of continuous standing. If it is possible to take a break and perform some stretching exercises throughout the day then this is highly recommended.

Evidence

As far as I am aware there have been no studies that have looked at rest as an isolated treatment option. However, anecdotally patients are often told to "rest" following advice from the GP with the understanding that the problem will self-resolve. Anecdotal evidence suggests that this is not the case and that rest as an isolated treatment option does not provide successful results in plantar fasciitis.

Risks

Boredom, frustration and possible weight gain due to reduced activity levels.

Verdict

As with any repetitive strain injury, relative rest is absolutely vital. In order to allow the strained fascia to heal it is necessary to reduce the loading stress or demand we are asking of it. A reduction in activity levels for a short period (usually a few weeks) whilst commencing other treatments encourages healing and a faster recovery. If relative rest is overlooked it can reduce your chances of healing despite the other treatment options such as stretching, orthoses, night splints etc.

Stretching Exercises

Rationale

The tightness of the Achilles tendon (the large tendon at the back of the lower leg) has long been implicated as a causative factor in plantar fasciitis. The main effect of having a tight Achilles tendon is reduced ankle joint range of motion, which results in abnormal loading stress on the foot. It is proven that a tight Achilles tendon will result in increased tensile stress on the plantar fascia, (Carlson et al 2000; Stecco 2013) therefore a logical treatment is to reduce this increased stress. This is easily achieved via stretching exercises which have long been prescribed to help treat plantar fasciitis. The positive clinical effect of stretching as a treatment regimen supports this theory (Davis et al 1994).

Evidence

Research has demonstrated a considerable association between limited ankle joint range of motion and plantar fasciitis. A recent study found that 211 of 254 (83%) patients with plantar fasciitis had limited ankle dorsiflexion (Patel & DiGiovanni 2011). Dorsiflexion is the movement which points the foot towards shin bone. However focusing stretching on the Achilles tendon only may provide suboptimal results. DiGiovanni and colleagues (2003) compared protocols of Achilles tendon stretching versus specific stretching of the plantar fascia. An Improvement was found in the plantar fascia stretch specific group at 8 weeks in 52% of patients, compared with 22% in the Achilles tendon only stretching group.

Porter et al (2002) conducted a prospective, randomised, blinded (moderate quality research) study. 94 patients (122 affected feet) were diagnosed with *"heel pain syndrome"*. patients were randomised into two stretching groups. One group performed sustained Achilles tendon stretches (three minutes, three times daily), the other performed intermittent stretches (five sets, 20 seconds each, two times daily). Participants were evaluated once a month for a period of four months. At each monthly visit, participants completed subjective questionnaires about their pain. Also, a physical therapist measured each participant's Achilles tendon flexibility.

The study determined that both groups had an increase in Achilles tendon flexibility. This increase in flexibility correlated with a decrease in pain. There was no significant difference in outcome between the sustained and intermittent stretching groups. The data suggest that both sustained and intermittent Achilles tendon stretching exercises were effective nonsurgical treatments for painful heel syndrome.

"heel pain syndrome" was defined in this study as plantar fasciitis, entrapment of the first branch of the lateral plantar nerve at the level of the abductor hallucis (muscle along the arch of the foot) and, possibly, the presence of a plantar heel spur. Meaning that the authors were not entirely sure what the true nature of the patient's symptoms was.

It has recently been found that patients are 8 times more likely to develop plantar fasciitis with tight hamstrings. The Labovitz et al (2011) study results indicate that an increase in hamstring tightness may induce prolonged forefoot loading and through the windlass mechanism (discussed later) be a factor that increases repetitive injury to the plantar fascia.

Another recent study also published in the medical journal - Foot & Ankle International also found a significant relationship between tight hamstrings as well in tight calf muscles in plantar fasciitis sufferers in comparison to a control group of people who did not have plantar fasciitis and who had good hamstring a calf flexibility (Bolivar et al 2013).

<u>Finally, the American Physical Therapy Association (APTA) published clinical practice guidelines for plantar fasciitis. They graded the overall evidence strength of different treatments ranging from A (highest strength) to F (lowest strength). Stretching exercises were graded as an A (APTA 2014).</u>

Risks

Soft tissue stretching exercises are generally very safe, low-risk treatment with no common associated risks providing they are done with the correct technique. If you experience any pain whilst performing any of these exercises you should discontinue them immediately and consult a podiatrist or suitable health professional.

Verdict

Poor flexibility of the Achilles tendon/posterior leg muscles (muscles at the back of the leg) is one of the main contributing factors to the development of plantar fasciitis due to the excess consequential mechanical overloading that occurs on the plantar fascia. There is also a good body of evidence to prove this association. Addressing tightness in the plantar fascia, Achilles tendon, calves and hamstrings (collectively known as the superficial back line) is perhaps the most important factor that must be addressed in the treatment of plantar fasciitis.

For detailed instructional videos on stretching exercises for the plantar fascia, calves, and hamstrings visit my youtube channel via the link below:

https://www.youtube.com/user/PlantarFasciitisGone

Night Splints

Rationale

Night splints offer a fantastically effortless way of preventing overnight tightness of the Achilles tendon and plantar fascia. During sleep, your feet naturally fall into a plantarflexed position. This means the feet are pointing downwards. This causes the calf muscles which are attached to the Achilles tendon to shorten and increases tension on the Achilles tendon which results in tightening of the plantar fascia.

When you awake and put your feet down to the ground to get out of bed the Achilles tendon and plantar fascia suddenly have to stretch back to the ankles neutral position in order for you to get your heel to make contact with the ground (otherwise you would be walking around on tip toes).

This rapid change in tendon and fascia length over such as short period causes micro-tearing of the plantar fascia which is why you get an immediate sharp, unrelenting pain response.

Because the night splint holds the ankle in its neutral position and pulls the toes backwards it does not allow the calf muscles or the plantar fascia to shorten overnight therefore when you put your feet down to the ground first thing in the morning the plantar fascia only has to stretch a minimal amount thus significantly reducing the pain and preventing damage.

Evidence

There have been a number of studies published looking at the effectiveness of night splints for plantar fasciitis which is detailed below:

The Journal of Foot and Ankle Surgery published a study in 2002 which compared 2 groups of patients with plantar fasciitis; group 1 wore a night splint but did not complete a stretching programme and group 2 only completed a stretching programme but did not wear a night splint.

Group 1 results – All but two of the patients treated with night splints recovered within 8 weeks (97.8%)

Group 2 results – only 57.7% of these patients that utilized the stretching protocol recovered within 8 weeks.

Conclusion – "The night splint treatment group had a significantly shorter recovery time compared to the stretching group" (Barry et al 2002).

It is noted that there were limitations to this study including adjunctive treatments and the use of pain as the only outcome measure

Another and recent study compared two different night splint designs:

- An anterior night splint - this means the material of the splint covers the front of the shin bone
- a posterior night splint - this means the material of the splints covers the calf muscle on the back of the leg

The results indicated that both night splints were effective at treating plantar fasciitis. The anterior night splint was found to be more effective in the treatment of plantar fasciitis. It was also proven to be better tolerated and more comfortable than the posterior night splint (Attard & Singh 2012).

A prospective randomised control trial (good quality research) was conducted by Roos et al (2006). They studied the effects of foot orthoses (insoles) and night splints, alone or combined, in a prospective, randomised trial with 1-year follow-up.

- Group 1 - orthoses and night splint (15 patients)
- Group 2 - orthoses only (13 patients)
- Group 3 - night splint only (15 patients)

The results demonstrated that at 12 weeks all groups improved significantly in all outcomes evaluated. There was a pain reduction of 30% to 50% compared to patients pain scores before treatment across all groups. At 1 year follow-up, pain reduction of 62% was seen in the two groups using orthoses compared to 48% in the night splint only group. In conclusion, the study found that orthoses and anterior night splints were effective both short-term and long-term in treating pain from plantar fasciitis. However, orthoses were better overall in the long term due to better compliance with this device.

Finally, the American Physical Therapy Association (APTA) published clinical practice guidelines for plantar fasciitis. They graded the overall evidence strength of different treatments ranging from A (highest strength) to F (lowest strength). night splints were graded as an A (APTA 2014).

Risks

The night splint is a safe treatment option for plantar fasciitis with no common associated risk. Ensure the night splint is fitted correctly and not fitted too tight to prevent adverse effects.

Verdict

In conclusion, there is moderate high-quality evidence to support the use of night splints in the management of plantar fasciitis. The night splint is an incredibly effective device at eliminating heel pain first thing in the morning which is what almost every patient with plantar fasciitis suffers with. The reasons for this are explained under the rationale section. The night splint is one of the most important treatment components for plantar fasciitis as it reduces damage to the plantar fascia when the patient gets out of bed in the morning. This breaks the pain cycle and promotes faster recovery time from plantar fasciitis.

Which is the best night splint?

This is dependent on patient preference. Most people find posterior night splints very bulky, uncomfortable and difficult to wear whilst sleeping. Posterior night splints have been shown to be less effective than anterior night splints are not recommended by the author. Anterior night splints are less bulky and more comfortable than posterior night splints. A limitation of the anterior night splint, however, is that it does not dorsiflex the toes, it only dorsiflexes the ankle joint. It has been clinically proven that dorsiflexion of the toes in combination with dorsiflexion of the ankle provides a maximum stretch on the plantar fascia and Achilles tendon (Carlson et al 2000; Flanigan 2007). The most recent night splint design, the sock design is not made from plastic and is the most comfortable of the three designs for most people. The sock design night splint provides dorsiflexion of the toes in a combination of dorsiflexion of the ankle, providing the most effective stretch whilst sleeping. Due to improved clinical effectiveness and improved comfort the sock design night splint is considered the best option.

Orthoses (Insoles)

Rationale

The most common cause cited in the medical literature for plantar fasciitis is the biomechanical stress of the plantar fascia, particularly at its attachment to the medial calcaneal tuberosity (heel bone). The main job role of the plantar fascia is to support the arch of the foot. The aim of insoles is to reduce the biomechanical stress placed on the plantar fascia by supporting the arch of the foot. Therefore it is no surprise that Insoles are amongst the most commonly reported treatment methods for plantar fasciitis.

Evidence

Campbell and Inman in 1974, were the first authors to describe success with mechanical therapy insoles. They treated 33 patients and retrospectively reported a 94% success rate.

Another study by O'Brien and Martin, in 1985, performed a retrospective telephone survey of 41 patients with 58 painful heels.

Excellent and good results were recorded for 96.7% of the patients, most of whom received multiple therapies. Subjectively, the patients stated that insoles were the most successful treatment modality.

It is noted that the two mentioned studies above a very dated and of poor quality

A more recently published study by Lynch et al (1998) concluded that mechanical control of the foot via insoles was more effective than anti-inflammatory therapy or accommodative therapy in the conservative treatment of plantar fasciitis.

The Roos et al (2006) study (referenced earlier in the night splints section) demonstrated that orthoses were effective for both short term and long term management of plantar fasciitis. This was a robust, good quality study.

Another randomised control trial (high-quality study) was conducted by Landorf and colleagues (2006). They compared 3 groups:

Group 1 custom made orthoses

Group 2 prefabricated orthoses

Group 3 Sham (fake) orthoses

Their findings were that foot orthoses produced small short-term benefits in function and small reductions in pain for people with plantar fasciitis. But they did not have long-term beneficial effects compared with a sham device. Meaning that at a 12-month review the foot orthoses were no better than a blank insole, essentially no treatment at all. There was no significant difference in effectiveness between the custom made orthoses and the prefabricated orthoses. So the small short-term pain relief seen in the two groups who had orthoses were very similar.

A cadaveric study (using donor's feet) was published by Kogler and colleagues (1995) to test the theory that orthoses do indeed support the arch of the foot as they are believed to. They measured the level of strain on the plantar fascia using an electromechanical test machine and applied a load to the foot whilst barefoot, in shoes and in different types of orthoses. They found that some of the orthoses (ones with better anti-pronation support) significantly reduced decreased strain in the plantar fascia compared with the barefoot condition. These study findings support the theory behind prescribing orthoses to reduce strain on the plantar fascia in the treatment of plantar fasciitis.

Finally, the American Physical Therapy Association (APTA) published clinical practice guidelines for plantar fasciitis. They graded the overall evidence strength of different treatments ranging from A (highest strength) to F (lowest strength). Stretching exercises were graded as an A (APTA 2014).

Risks

The use of Insoles is generally a very safe treatment option and is commonly prescribed to help with a large array of musculoskeletal conditions including plantar fasciitis.

A small percentage of people experience adverse effects from wearing insoles which may include blistering of the skin on the sole of the foot, aches, and pains in other joints such as knee, hips and lower back. Most of these aches and pains subside once you become used to your insoles which usually takes approximately 1-2 weeks. Wearing insoles should not cause acute pain. If you experience pain as a result of wearing insoles you should stop wearing them immediately and seek advice from a podiatrist.

Verdict

Insoles play a vital role in the multi-faceted approach to treating plantar fasciitis. Like stretching exercises, insoles help address and reduce the mechanical stress that leads to injury of the plantar fascia as has been proven in cadaveric studies. There is a good level of high-quality evidence to prove their efficacy in the treatment of plantar fasciitis both in short and long term and are therefore considered an evidence-based treatment option.

Massage Roller

Rationale

Massage involves the manipulation of superficial and deeper layers of muscle and connective tissue, to enhance function, aid in the healing process, and promote relaxation and well-being.

When there is chronic soft tissue tension injury, there are usually adhesions (bands of painful, rigid tissue). These adhesions can cause pain, limited movement, and inflammation. Deep tissue massage works by physically breaking down these adhesions to relieve pain and restore normal movement

Evidence

Despite its popularity, there is a lack of evidence to support massage therapy as a treatment option for musculoskeletal injuries in isolation.

On the other hand, there is recent evidence to suggest that massage can play an anti-inflammatory role and aid healing in soft tissue injuries in a similar way to that of nonsteroidal anti-inflammatory drugs such as ibuprofen (Crane et al 2012).

Risks

A massage roller is a safe therapeutic treatment option to aid healing of plantar fasciitis.

Verdict

Massage therapy in isolation is unlikely to heal plantar fasciitis in the long term as this treatment does not address the underlying mechanical cause of the condition. It does, however, provide a therapeutic benefit to the patient and complements other mechanical treatment modalities to aid the healing the process.

Footwear Modification

Rationale

There is an all too common link between poor, unsupportive footwear and plantar fasciitis. Unfortunately, this is largely due to the modern shoe industry which focuses their shoe designs on fashion purposes instead of what is supportive for a person's feet. Shoes should have adequate arch support and cushioned heels. Worn or ill-fitting shoes can exacerbate plantar fasciitis due to lack of proper support and cushion.

Evidence

As far as I am are aware currently there have been no studies to investigate the effectiveness of footwear change in the treatment of plantar fasciitis, however, an interesting case report published in a medical journal The Foot highlighted the importance of suitable footwear.

A patient presented with bilateral (both heels) plantar fasciitis with a 1-month onset. Following a footwear assessment, it was noted that the inner material in the heel of the shoes was excessively worn.

A simple footwear change to the new shoes with no other treatment method applied, fully resolved the pain after 4 weeks (Rajput & Abboud 2004). This study suggests that footwear is often overlooked as a causative factor in the development of plantar fasciitis and is an independent causative factor of plantar fasciitis.

Risks

The only risk here is your fashion status. Most shoes that are considered supportive and helpful for plantar fasciitis aren't considered 'fashionable' with today's trends.

Verdict

The importance of suitable footwear is paramount in the success of treating plantar fasciitis. Unsuitable footwear can affect the effectiveness of treatment or prolong the condition, which might be alleviated otherwise. This advice is particularly stressed towards female patients as their footwear choices are usually worse than men's. Shoes which often make plantar fasciitis worse are flat slip on shoes or pumps. Ugg boots are also very bad. Flip flops are bad unless there is an arch contour built into the bed of the flip-flop to provide some arch support. Avoid shoes with a no or a low heel. This does not mean you have the live out the rest of your days in "ugly shoes". The aim of wearing supportive shoes is to reduce strain on the plantar fascia and avoid aggravating the condition. Once the plantar fascia is healed one may return to unsupportive footwear gradually and monitor their symptoms. For some people, they will be lucky enough to go back to wearing whatever shoe they please. Unfortunately, others may have to be a bit more sensible with their footwear options. There is no way of predicting this. The take home message here is that footwear choice is just as important as all the other treatment components and is not to be overlooked.

See my available video on basic footwear advice and recommendations

https://www.youtube.com/watch?v=iKy7qhAzg04

Extra-corporeal Shockwave Therapy (ESWT)

Rationale

shockwave therapy is a relatively new technology used to treat chronic (long-term) soft tissue disease such as plantar fasciitis that has failed to respond to normal treatment. The technology is based on lithotripsy, which has been used for many years to treat kidney stones. High-energy sound waves are created and focused on the injury using a special applicator. Shockwaves are repeatedly applied to the injury area, which breaks down scar tissue and calcifications in the area. The body's own natural healing capacity will usually fulfill this role however in chronic cases the body is sometimes unable to repair itself. As the shockwave breaks down the tissue, it re-induces the acute phase of healing and so the body starts generating new tissue leading to healing. It's like giving your body a second chance to heal itself.

Evidence

Current research has demonstrated positive outcomes in terms of pain relief and quality of life measures (Lee et al 2003; Malay et al 2006; Gollwitzer et al 2007; Chuckpaiwong et al 2009). Another study has demonstrated a decrease in plantar fascia thickness under ultrasound examination after ESWT (Androsoni et al 2013). Furthermore, a recent systematic review supported the use of ESWT for plantar fasciitis treatment (Speed 2012). On the other hand, there are studies which have failed to demonstrate a difference between ESWT and placebo (Buchbinder 2002; Marks et al 2008).

The National Institute for Health and Care Excellence (NICE), which provides national UK guidance believe that the current evidence on its efficacy is inconsistent. However, it should be pointed out that their guidance was last updated in 2009 and since then further research has been provided supporting the use of ESWT. Furthermore NICE made this statement due to a large diversity in treatment protocols including; the technology used to administer shockwaves, the number of treatment sessions, the time interval between treatment

sessions, as well as the option to administer local anaesthesia which has been reported to influence the outcome of shockwave therapy. NICE Guidance does not recommend a specific number sessions stating 'between one and several.' The guidance also reports different energies can be used. Finally, NICE recommends that clinicians conduct audit and review clinical outcomes for all patients having ESWT for refractory plantar fasciitis

An interesting study noted the irrelevance of heel spurs when treating plantar fasciitis with ESWT. In a large prospective study by Lee et al (2003) consisting of 435 patients with chronic proximal plantar fasciitis, 283 (65%) had an inferior calcaneal bone spur of variable size evident prior to treatment with high-energy ESWT. This included 308 patients who received extracorporeal shockwave treatments and 127 placebo patients. At both initial (3 months) and final (12 months) evaluations after receiving ESWT, no patient who received shock wave applications had significant disappearance or change in the X-ray appearance of the heel spur. Clinical outcome after ESWT was satisfactory in 168 patients (82%) with a demonstrable heel spur on x-ray and in 81 patients (79%) without such a heel spur. The results showed no correlation between the presence or absence of the heel spur and the eventual treatment outcome. In essence, the presence or absence of a heel spur did not matter.

The latest evidence for ESWT is very promising with around 75% success rate in chronic plantar fasciitis that has failed to respond to usual treatment including stretching, footwear modifications, insoles.

Risks

Generally, ESWT is very safe. It is non-invasive and does not require a local anaesthetic. Common risks include a potential for hemorrhage and local soft tissue damage which may lead to bruising. Patients on anticoagulant treatment (blood thinners) will need to stop their medication before receiving shockwave therapy due to increased risk of bleeding. It is advised to seek medical advice if you are considering ESWT.

Verdict

ESWT is an excellent treatment option for chronic cases (longer than 3 months) of plantar fasciitis. In the author's experience, over 70% of cases are chronic before patients decide to seek treatment. This is often due to patients ignoring their initial symptoms in the hope that the pain will self-resolve waiting to be referred to see a podiatrist before starting treatment. This often means that the degenerative changes within the plantar fascia are more advanced and are less likely to heal despite normal treatment. This is when ESWT is an excellent treatment option to repair tissue degeneration and kick start the healing process. However, it should not be used as an isolated treatment as it does not address the underlying cause of the condition. ESWT increased your body's own ability to heal itself and should, therefore, be used as an adjunctive treatment with other mechanical treatments such as stretching, orthoses, night splint, and footwear modification.

Shockwave therapy is proven to be as effective as traditional surgery and doesn't involve an operation, being in plaster, or a long rehabilitation period which can last over 6 months. Shockwave therapy only requires one treatment weekly over 3-4 weeks. Treatment is safe, non-invasive, only takes 10 minutes and is as good as results achieved by surgery.

Weight Loss

Rationale

It is a logical assumption that the higher a person's total body weight (body mass index), the higher the peak pressure placed on the foot as this is the body's main weight bearing support structure. This excessive peak pressure placed on the heel is believed to be a primary intrinsic risk factor for the development of plantar fasciitis, with a large body of scientific evidence to support this claim as displayed below.

Evidence

Research supports the logical assumption above by demonstrating that obese adults experience higher plantar pressures in comparison to non-obese adults (Hills et al 2001). One study observed that individuals with a body mass index (BMI) > 30 kg/m had an odds ratio of 5.6 for PF compared to those with a BMI < 25 kg/m2 (Riddle et al 2005). Another study consisting of 1411 patients found that being overweight or obese significantly increased the chances of having tendinitis in general. If the person were overweight or obese, there was an increased likelihood of plantar fasciitis (Frey & Zamora 2007). There is an additional explanation for the link between high BMI and plantar fasciitis, Faria et al (2009) found that as body mass index increases, muscle-tendon unit stiffness also increases. This suggests that people with a higher BMI will have an increased risk of a tight Achilles tendon which as we know, increases the risk of developing plantar fasciitis.

Verdict

If you are overweight and suffer from plantar fasciitis it is of paramount importance that you include weight loss as part of your treatment plan. Ignoring this simple component may prevent a person from gaining the most out of their treatment as carrying excess weight is linked to plantar fasciitis. Weight loss can be achieved in a number of ways. Amongst the most effective are diet and exercise. Understandably, this is easier said than done however there are many weight loss programmes readily available that can help you achieve this.

With regards to exercise as a weight loss method, I recommend low-impact activities such as cycling, using a cross trainer or rowing machine or swimming as these will not cause impact related pain to the heel. Running, particularly on a hard surface not recommended and may worsen your plantar fasciitis as it is a high impact activity.

Strengthening exercises

Rationale

Strengthening exercises are often overlooked in the conventional treatment of plantar fasciitis. This may be due to the notion that strengthening exercises may place further strain on the plantar fascia and worsen the condition. This notion, to a degree, may hold some truth and it is therefore not recommended to perform strengthening exercises in the acute phase of the treatment plan. However, by having weak plantarflexors, for example, the calf muscles, may cause an abnormal gait (walking) because weakened muscles have diminished force absorption and production capabilities. Therefore increased compensatory stress may be placed on other structures, which can lead to force overload on the plantar fascia, tissue microtrauma, and pain.

Evidence

There is evidence to demonstrate an association of weak plantarflexor muscles with plantar fasciitis and other foot disorders (Kibler et al 1991). Although it is not known if the strength deficits are present before injury or whether they are caused secondary to the condition. The authors of this study concluded that a strength deficit of the posterior calf is present in the foot suffering from plantar fasciitis, which creates a functional deficit in the normal foot biomechanics. This deficit either contributes or causes to overt clinical symptoms and should be addressed in the evaluation and treatment of plantar fasciitis.

An exciting recent Scandinavian study (Rathleff et al 2014) compared strengthening exercises vs. plantar fascia stretching exercises in 48 patients with ultrasound scan confirmed plantar fasciitis. Patients were randomised into two groups:

group 1 - strengthening exercises and gel heel cup (24 patients)

group 2 - plantar fascia stretching exercises and gel heel cup (24 patients)

At a 3 month follow-up, the strengthening exercise group demonstrated significantly less foot pain in comparison with the plantar fascia stretch group. However, a 6 month and 12-month review did not demonstrate a difference between to two groups with both improving overall. It is important to highlight that there were no differences seen on ultrasound scan follow-up between the two groups with both demonstrating reduced thickening of the plantar fascia. In conclusion, the strength exercise group made quicker improvements which leveled by 6 and 12 months.

Why was the strength training associated with superior improvement?

What we know is that high-load strength training that causes controlled high tensile loads across a tendon has shown promising results on degenerative tendon disorders such as Achilles and patellar tendinopathy. Although fascia is not the same as tendon they are similar as both are made up of type 1 collagen fibres (Stecco et al 2013). It appears that this type of collagen responds to high-load through increased collagen synthesis (Langberg et al 2007). As patients with plantar fasciitis show degenerative changes at the plantar fascia enthesis (Jarde et al 2003; Lemont et al 2003), increased collagen synthesis may help normalise fascia structure and improve pain.

Risks

Soft tissue strengthening exercises are generally a very safe, low-risk treatment with no common associated risks providing they are done with the correct technique. It is possible one may overwork a muscle by doing too much of their stretching exercises and over exert themselves. It is therefore advised that you introduce the exercises regime with a modest start with very gradual progression. If you experience any pain whilst performing the strengthening exercises you discontinue them immediately and consult a podiatrist or suitably qualified health professional.

Verdict

Strengthening exercises certainly do play a role in the treatment plan for plantar fasciitis. The question is when? At current there is a lack of agreement as to when to introduce these exercises as loading the plantar fascia at the wrong stage may worsen pain, however, this did not appear to be the case in the recent Rathleff et al study (2014). It is recommended to perform calf strengthening exercises whilst symptoms have settled with the aim preventing recurrence of plantar fasciitis as strengthening exercises will improve posterior calf muscle strength and help optimise gait (walking).

Similar to stretching exercises, there are a number of different techniques available to strengthen the posterior calf muscles. My available video (see link below) teaches you how to perform these exercises with the correct technique and more importantly how not to perform them, as unfortunately many patients develop bad technique habits after being shown how to perform their strengthening exercises or after following written instructions on a leaflet.

https://www.youtube.com/watch?v=e1Ocwox6S9A&t=1s

Taping

Rationale

Taping is one method that has been utilised to biomechanically control tensile forces generated through the plantar fascia (Saxelby 1997). The concept of taping of the foot to treat plantar fasciitis is by reducing foot pronation which has been linked with increased tensile stress on the plantar fascia (Cornwall & McPoil 1999). It is an alternative to foot orthoses (insoles).

Evidence

There is limited high-quality research to support the effectiveness of taping for plantar fasciitis. Saxelby and colleagues (1997) found a significant improvement in symptoms with the use of taping, however, the study group was very small (9 participants) and was only tested over two days. A recent study was conducted looking at the biomechanical effect of taping at reducing medial arch collapse. It was demonstrated that there are measurable changes to medial arch height and amount of arch height deformation during gait following low-Dye taping (the most common technique used). Although changes were present immediately after application, results were diminished 48 hours after application. The most likely explanation for this is the material fatigue of the tape after 48 hours. Finally a recent systematic review regarding the efficacy of taping concluded – There is limited evidence that taping can reduce pain in the short term in patients with plantar fasciitis (Van de Water & Speknijder 2010).

Risks

Taping is generally considered a safe treatment if shown how to apply the tape safely by a suitable health professional. The incorrect taping technique can lead to blistering of the skin. Too much tension applied by the tape could lead constriction of the blood vessels in the foot and ankle leading to ischaemia (reduced blood supply). This risk is further increased in diabetic patients who often suffer from reduced blood supply to the feet and neuropathy (lack of protective sensation).

Verdict

Taping can improve plantar fasciitis symptoms in the short term. However, mastering a correct taping technique for self-application is not an easy task and is deemed impractical as a self-care treatment in the long term. There is some evidence to suggest taping is effective at reducing plantar fasciitis symptoms but only as a short-term effect. In order for taping to work in the long term, it would require the patient to continue to tape their foot over months on a daily basis. More importantly due to the limited existing supportive evidence on taping as an effective treatment for plantar fasciitis, I do not value the usage of taping as a treatment option. Currently, there is no consensus of what taping technique is the most effective.

Corticosteroid Injections

Rationale

Corticosteroid injections are a common short-term treatment for plantar fasciitis. They are usually injected at the source of pain, the attachment of the plantar fascia to the heel bone. The aim of a steroid injection is to reduce inflammation and thickening of the fascia and reduce pain shortly after the injection.

Evidence

Currently, there is some evidence to suggest that corticosteroids are good for short term relief but there is no evidence to support the use of steroid injections as a long-term treatment option. Indeed, a recent study found that ultrasound-guided corticosteroid injection was significantly better than placebo at four weeks post-injection however it was no better at 8 weeks or 12 weeks (McMillan et al 2012). One of the reasons for this is that a steroid injection does not address the underlying cause of the problem; it merely serves as a temporary pain relief.

Risks

Steroid injections come with their risks. Firstly, as with most injections, steroid injections are a painful experience. Corticosteroid infiltration has been found to predispose the plantar fascia to rupture, however, there is a lack of consensus as to how significant the risk is but it is reported to be around 5% of cases where patients have received at least 2 injections. A corticosteroid injection can also cause the heel fat bad to become thinner, which means the heel has less fat pad available to aid in shock absorption (Sellman 1994).

In a review article on the treatment options for plantar fasciitis Roxas concluded: *"Corticosteroid injections provide temporary relief from pain and are recommended only in extreme cases, as they may increase the risk of infection and contribute to further degeneration of the plantar fascia and heel fat pad"* (Roxas 2005).

Verdict

Not recommended.

In light of recent evidence that plantar fasciitis is more accurately defined as plantar fasciosis, which is a degenerative condition as opposed to an inflammatory condition the indication of a corticosteroid injection which is a potent anti-inflammatory agent is questionable. There is no doubt that corticosteroid injections do help with pain relief in the short term however this treatment does not address the underlying cause of the problem and should, therefore, always be used as an adjunctive treatment along with other treatments such as stretches, night splints, orthoses, suitable footwear and weight loss.

Therapeutic Ultrasound

Rationale

There are a number of reported benefits of therapeutic ultrasound when used for musculoskeletal conditions. Firstly, is the speeding up of the healing process from the increase in blood flow to the injured area. Secondly, is the decrease in pain from the reduction of swelling and oedema. Thirdly, is the gentle massage of muscles, tendons and/ or ligaments in the treated area because no strain is added and any scar tissue is softened.

Evidence

Despite the rather attractive claims of therapeutic ultrasound, unfortunately, there is very limited evidence that therapeutic ultrasound is more effective than placebo ultrasound for treating people with pain or a range of musculoskeletal injuries or for promoting soft tissue healing (Baker et al 2001).

A systematic review conducted by Windt et al (1999) concluded:

*"As yet, there seems to be **little evidence to support the use of ultrasound therapy** in the treatment of musculoskeletal disorders. The large majority of 13 randomized placebo-controlled trials with adequate methods **did not support the existence** of clinically important or statistically significant differences in favour of ultrasound therapy."*

Risks

Therapeutic ultrasound is generally a safe treatment option. There is a potential risk of overheated bodily tissues if used for long duration or high dose. In the hands of a qualified clinician, this risk is minimal.

Verdict

Amongst the most common treatment options available for plantar fasciitis, therapeutic ultrasound has perhaps the weakest evidence base for its efficacy. At best, ultrasound may increase blood flow to the injured area which may aid healing of plantar fasciitis. It is not considered an evidence-based treatment, is certainly not cost effective, and is not a recommended treatment for plantar fasciitis

Acupuncture

Rationale

Acupuncture has been used for many musculoskeletal pain conditions, including heel pain. A number of mechanisms have been proposed to explain the pain-relieving effect of acupuncture, including central opioid pain inhibition, diffuse noxious inhibitory control (DNIC) system and anti-inflammation. Presumably, insertion of a needle at any part of the body may alleviate pain by the mechanisms of opioids or DNIC, and the anti-inflammatory action of acupuncture may be generalized across the body.

Evidence

There is a lack of evidence to support the use of acupuncture, however, a randomised control trial of acupuncture for the treatment of plantar fasciitis was conducted by Zhang et al (2011). The study compared two different needling techniques: The treatment group (28 participants) received needling at the acupoint PC 7, which is purported to have a specific effect on heel pain. The control group (25 participants) received needling at the acupoint Hegu (LI 4), which has analgesic properties. In the treatment, they found a 40% reduction of morning pain at 1-month follow-up, which would be of significance to the patient. The control group demonstrated no improvement, however. A limitation of this study was that the authors were not able to assess the efficacy of the intended acupuncture treatment compared with placebo. Therefore it is uncertain whether the positive effects of acupuncture were a result of the specific needling technique, a placebo effect, or a combination of both.

Risks

When conducted by a qualified practitioner acupuncture is safe. Mild, short-lasting side effects occur in around 7-11% of patients. These include:

- Pain where the needles puncture the skin
- bleeding or bruising where the needles puncture the skin
- drowsiness
- worsening of pre-existing symptoms

Serious complications from treatment, such as infections or damage to tissue, are extremely rare. They usually occur only as a result of bad practice, carried out by an acupuncturist who has not been properly trained.

Verdict

The available evidence suggests that acupuncture may have positive anti-inflammatory effects on plantar fasciitis pain in the short term. However, there is no evidence to suggest it is any more effective than conventional anti-inflammatories including nonsteroidal anti-inflammatory medication such as ibuprofen. This treatment method like other reported anti-inflammatory treatments may compliment healing; however, it should not be relied on as a long-term resolution to plantar fasciitis as it does not address the underlying cause of plantar fasciitis. Acupuncture is not considered an evidence-based or cost effective treatment.

Immobilisation

Rationale

Immobilisation is less frequently used as a conventional treatment for plantar fasciitis in comparison to stretching exercises, insoles etc, possibly because it is less practical to completely immobilise the foot. Instead, mobilisation is reserved for use in recalcitrant (nonresponsive) cases that have failed to respond to conventional treatments.

Evidence

As far as I am aware there have been no studies investigating the efficacy of foot immobilisation as a treatment option for plantar fasciitis.

Risks

Increased risk of deep vein thrombosis (blood clot) due to prolonged immobilisation. Decreased muscle tone and shrinkage of the lower limb muscles (atrophy). There is the possibility of decreased circulation if the cast fits too tightly. Excessive pressure over a nerve (most likely the common peroneal nerve) can cause irritation or possible damage if not corrected.

Verdict

Immobilisation may play a role in the treatment of plantar fasciitis in chronic cases that have failed conservative treatment based on the theory that whilst the foot is immobilised the plantar fascia will not be under weight bearing stress thus allowing it to heal. It should be considered before surgical intervention. Anecdotally is it often reported that patients experience significant pain relief during and immediately after cast immobilisation, however, symptoms often return after 1 month. Once a patient has immobilised the foot for 4-6 weeks to allow healing this should be followed up with a careful rehabilitation programme to prevent recurrence of the condition.

Platelet Rich Plasma (PRP) Injections

Rationale

Platelet Rich Plasma (PRP) injections are a relatively new treatment that involves taking a patient's own blood (usually from the arm) and placing the blood into a special machine (centrifuge) to separate different components of the blood. This allows the clinician to use concentrated levels of platelets and growth factors found in the blood sample which is then injected at the site of injury to promote healing in injured plantar fascia tissue. Regarding the way in which PRP works, some laboratory studies have demonstrated that the increased concentration of growth factors in PRP are able to augment the body's natural healing process

Evidence

A recent level 1 study (high quality) compared PRP injections with corticosteroid injections. Both treatments demonstrated good results at 3 months however the corticosteroid group returned to baseline levels of pain at 12 months whilst the PRP still demonstrated significant pain relief at 12 months and also at 24 months following treatment (Monto 2014). There are a number of other recent studies which have demonstrated PRP to be superior to corticosteroid injections (Shetty et al 2014; Akashin et al 2012).

Below is a conclusion from a recent systematic review (Franceschi et al 2014).

"Evidence for the use of PRP in PF shows promising results, and this therapy appears safe. However, the number of studies available is limited and randomized placebo-controlled studies are required. Characterizing the details of the intervention and standardizing the outcome scores would help to better document the responses and optimize the treatment."

Risks

PRP is not generally considered to have any major harmful effects because apart from a patient's own blood, no other constituents are added to the injection. For that reason, it is popular with patients who want more of a 'natural approach' to dealing with their injuries. There is a small risk of infection as with any injection therapy.

Verdict

The theory behind PRP injection therapy makes this an attractive treatment option for chronic plantar fasciitis that has not responded to usual conservative treatment. There is a lack of high-quality evidence at this stage to be sure on the true efficacy of this treatment option. For now, this remains a 'watch this space' treatment and certainly an option worth considering before surgical intervention as it is less invasive and comes with minimal risks.

Botulinum Toxin A (Botox) Injections

Rationale

Botulinum toxin A (Botox) injections were originally used to treat neurological conditions resulting in spastic paralysis (stiffening of muscles) such as cerebral palsy. It has more recently been employed for the treatment of musculoskeletal conditions including plantar fasciitis. Botox injections are used to relax muscles and other soft tissue. As it is widely accepted that tightness in the calf muscles is a causative factor in plantar fasciitis, Botox injections aim to relax contracture (tightening) in these muscles thus reducing tensile strain on the plantar fascia as a result of muscle relaxation. The mechanism of action of this toxin involves blocking the release of acetylcholine at the neuromuscular junctions resulting in flaccid paralysis

Evidence

A level 1, double-blinded, randomised control trial (good quality study) compared Botox vs. Corticosteroid injection for treatment of plantar fasciitis (Elizondo-Rodriguez et al 2013).

Group 1 - Botox injection and plantar fascia stretching (19 patients)

Group 1 - corticosteroid injection and plantar fascia stretching (17 patients)

Results were recorded at 2 weeks, 1, 2, 4, and 6 months. There were no significant improvements in either group after the initial 2-week review. Both groups showed significant improvements in pain scores at 1 month. At the 2, 4 and 6 months follow up the Botox group had significantly better scores than the steroid group. At the final 6 month review the average pain score for the Botox group was 1.1/10 reduced from 7.1/10 (difference = 6) and 3.8/10 reduced from 7.7/10 (difference = 3.9) in the steroid group.

This study found that Botox injections were a superior treatment option than corticosteroid injections for the treatment of plantar fasciitis for short-term and mid-term (Elizondo-Rodriguez et al 2013). A limitation of this study is that patients were not followed up over a longer period (at least 12 months) which would inform us whether Botox is also successful in long-term management for plantar fasciitis.

A similar study compared Botox injections with corticosteroid injections. This study was also a randomised control trial with 28 patients in each group. Like the Elizondo-Rodriquez study (2013) they found both Botox and corticosteroid injections successful at the 1-month review, however, the difference between the two treatments became larger at 6 months with the Botox group continuing to improve whilst the steroid group got slightly worse (Diaz-Llopis et al 2012).

Diaz-Llopis followed up their original study in 2012. They conducted a 12 month follow up in the Botox group to see if they had sustained improvements in the long term which they did. This provides evidence to support the use of Botox as a long-term treatment option (Diaz-Llopis et al 2013).

A study by Babcock et al (2005) compared Botox injections with placebo. This was a double-blinded, randomised, placebo-controlled study in 27 patients with plantar fasciitis. The results were recorded 3 weeks and 8 weeks and observed significant changes in the Botox group compared to the placebo-controlled group. A limitation of this study is the short term follow up.

Another study found Botox injections to be superior to placebo in a double-blind, randomised control trial of 50 patients (25 each group). They found Botox to be significantly better than placebo at 1 month and 6-month reviews. The Botox group also showed significant reduction in plantar fascia thickness which demonstrates healing of the degenerative plantar fascia. This was not seen in the control group. A further benefit of Botox is that it did not reduce heel fat pad thickness which is a commonly reported complication with steroid injections.

On the other hand a similar study compared Botox injections with placebo, however, they found only marginal differences between the two groups. 63.1% of the Botox group perceived an improvement versus 55% of the placebo group (Peterlein et al 2012).

Risks

Botox injections are generally a safe treatment and major side effects are uncommon when administered in the hands of a suitably qualified clinician.

Although very unlikely, there is a possibility that the effect of botulinum toxin may spread to other parts of the body and cause botulism-like signs and symptoms. Call your doctor right away if you notice any of these effects hours to weeks after receiving Botox:

- Muscle weakness all over the body
- Vision problems
- Trouble speaking or swallowing
- Trouble breathing
- Loss of bladder control

Verdict

Overall it would appear that the current evidence base on Botox injections for treatment of plantar fasciitis is sufficient to support its use. Most studies of moderate to high quality demonstrate significant success with this treatment option. Despite this Botox injections are not a common treatment option and are not widely available for treating this condition, not at least in the UK and is something which deserves greater attention for clinical practice.

Trigger Point Therapy

Rationale

Trigger point therapy has become increasingly popular over recent years in the UK and is currently the hot topic for relieving a wide range of musculoskeletal pain including plantar fasciitis. Trigger point therapy has been around since 1942 where it was first coined by Dr. J Travell following her work on myofascial pain syndrome. Myofascial pain syndrome is described as hyperirritable areas associated within a taut band of a skeletal muscle that is painful on compression, contraction, or stretching of the muscles, and elicit a referred pain distant to the trigger point (Simons et al 1999). It is believed that trigger point therapy allows your body to undergo soft tissue release, allowing for increased blood flow, a reduction in muscle spasm, and the break-up of scar tissue. It is also believed to help remove any build-up of toxic metabolic waste.

Evidence

Although there is considerable anecdotal evidence, currently there is a paucity of clinical research evidence to support the use of trigger point therapy, however, one particular study looked at trigger point therapy in the management of plantar fasciitis.

A randomized clinical control trial compared two groups of patients - trigger point therapy and stretching vs. stretching alone. Patients receiving a combination of self-stretching and Trigger point therapy intervention showed a greater improvement in pressure pain thresholds, as compared to those who received only the self-stretching protocol (Renen-Ordine et al 2011).

Risks

Trigger point therapy is generally a safe treatment option if carried out correctly. Before self-treating, with trigger point therapy one should be screened by a suitably qualified health professional to assess whether it is safe to administer this treatment. Or at least follow an instructional DVD to minimise harmful effects. Trigger point therapy may not be suitable for people who have circulatory problems such as a history of DVT (blood clot) due to the risk of vessel damage and movement of any clot which can result in a serious life threatening emergency.

Verdict

Regardless of whether myofascial pain syndrome truly exists or whether there are specific trigger points within the body or not, trigger point therapy can be used effectively as an additional method to loosen tight calf muscles. They are an excellent adjunct along with a traditional stretching programme to make further gains in flexibility and a speedier recovery from plantar fasciitis. As this is a simple and safe treatment it is highly recommended.

Radiotherapy

Rationale

Radiation therapy has been used for at least 60 years because of its known anti-inflammatory effect. However, the exact mechanism is still unknown. Recent experiments show that low doses of radiation can modulate a variety of inflammation processes and the function of cellular components believed to be beneficial in treating chronic inflammation and degenerative diseases (Niewald et al 2012; Badakhshi & Buadch 2014).

Evidence

A prospective, randomized trial was initiated comparing the analgesic effect of a standard dose of radiotherapy (6 Gy) with that of a low dose (0.6 Gy), which proved with a high level of evidence the necessity of such a standard dose (Niewald et al 2012). There was a clear superiority of the standard dose (6 Gy) over the low-dose (0.6 Gy) concerning pain relief as well as quality of life (Niewald et al 2012).

Heyd et al (2007) randomised 130 patients between low-dose (LD) radiotherapy (3.0 Gy in 6 fractions over 3 weeks) and high-dose (HD) radiotherapy (6.0 Gy in 6 fractions over 3 weeks). If there was insufficient pain response then a second course of treatment was administered. Before treatment, 90.8% had severe pain and 9.8% had moderate pain. Six weeks after radiotherapy there was a response in 80% in the LD group and 84.6% in the HD group. Toxicity was minimal, with 28% experiencing a slight increase in pain during radiotherapy. Overall, at six-month follow-up, 87.7% had an improvement in pain, with no significant difference between the two groups.

Risks

The risk of radiation-induced cancer after radiotherapy for plantar fasciitis will be similar to that estimated for Dupuytren's disease (0.02%) since the doses and age range are similar (see section on Dupuytren's disease). This estimate is based on a field size of 60cm^2 so this should be taken into account if the field is larger or smaller. The risk decreases with increasing age at treatment. As a matter of course patients should be counseled as to the risk of radiation-induced cancer, which should be more strongly emphasized in younger patients.

The risk of other cancers outside the irradiated field, assuming adequate shielding for the remaining parts of the body, should be small due to the location of the radiation field at the extremity of the leg. Other possible consequences of radiation exposure at the recommended dose will be similar to those indicated for Dupuytren's disease.

Verdict

Radiotherapy appears to be an effective treatment based on the limited available evidence which is of high quality. Radiotherapy may be considered for patients who have had plantar fasciitis for more than six months and who have failed conservative management. This type of treatment is not available through the NHS in the UK and is not widely provided in the private sector. If you are interested in radiotherapy for plantar fasciitis you can find more information here on where you can receive this treatment - www.thedupuytrenspractice.com

Surgery

Rationale

In terms of treatment pathways, surgery has long been considered a last resort treatment for plantar fasciitis (Thomas et al 2010). This is largely due to the high success rate (approximately 90%) of conservative (non-surgical) treatment. However, in the other 10% of patient's, surgery is occasionally carried out. The idea is that surgical plantar fascia release may provide relief of focal stress and therefore should relieve associated heel pain.

Evidence

There is indeed evidence that reports symptomatic relief following surgery (Barrett et al 1995). There are a countless number of procedures a surgeon may carry out to manage plantar fasciitis which makes it difficult to support or refute its success rate, as each outcome will be dependent on the specific procedure carried out. This is further complicated by the characteristics of the individual patient. Currently, there is insufficient data or high-quality research that exists to support the various surgical procedures available for use in the surgical treatment of plantar fasciitis.

Risks

Surgery is invasive and most procedures come with a lengthy recovery period. There is no guarantee that surgery will relieve the pain. Common reported problems following surgery include; stress fractures, lateral column pain (pain on the outside of the foot), acquired flat foot, and midfoot arthritis (Huang et al 1993; Robert et al 2000). The reason for these complications following surgery is due to the integral support the plantar fascia provides to the architecture of the foot. If the plantar fascia is released via surgical excision this releases the plantar fascia of its job, which can lead to collapse of the foot thus secondary complications as listed above.

Verdict

It is difficult to conclude whether surgery is a good or bad option for plantar fasciitis mainly because there are so many different procedures, some of which will be better suited for some patients whilst other procedures may be better suited for other patients. If one is going to have surgery to treat plantar fasciitis then it is of absolutely paramount importance that the surgeon carefully chooses the most appropriate procedure for that individual patient and that all evidence based non-surgical options have been explored. This ensures that surgery is the right option and will improve the chances of a successful post-op result.

Chapter Five

Heel Pain Differential Diagnoses: Other Causes of Heel Pain

Heel Pain of Neural Origin

Heel pain of a neural origin can be a debilitation condition for sufferers and may play a role in both acute and chronic heel pain. It may present as an isolated entity or it may present secondary to chronic plantar fasciitis and it can often be very difficult to differentiate between plantar fascia pain and neural pain. The first report of heel pain of a neural origin was published in a Dutch language article by Roegholt in 1940. To date, although nerve entrapment in plantar heel pain is well documented (e.g. Baxter and Pfeffer, 1992; Oztuna et al., 2002), its pathophysiology, diagnosis and management are still subject to debate.

There are a number of nerves in the foot which present as pain due to entrapment of the nerve.

Entrapment of Baxter's Nerve (1st Branch of the lateral plantar nerve)

Baxter's nerve entrapment is reported to be the most common cause of heel pain of neural origin. Baxter's nerve is the first branch of the lateral plantar nerve (1st B-LPN). Dissection studies have reported a site of possible entrapment between the abductor hallucis and the medial head of quadratus plantae muscle (Rondhuis & Huson 1986). Histological (microscopical) examination of this nerve revealed abnormal findings, suggesting chronic compression of the nerve (Baxter and Pfeffer 1992).

Entrapment of the Medial Calcaneal Nerve

The medial calcaneal nerve provides sensation to most of the heel fat pad and to the superficial tissues overlying the inferior part of the calcaneus. Entrapment of the medial calcaneal nerve is the second most commonly reported nerve that has been related to plantar heel pain of neural origin. However, entrapment of the medial calcaneal nerve may not be a very prevalent condition as only 5 out of 200 surgical cases were consistent with MCN entrapment (Schon et al 1993). Most branches of the Medial calcaneal nerve lie superficially to the abductor hallucis, flexor digitorum brevis and plantar fascia (Arenson et al 1980; Louisia and Masquelet, 1999) and are therefore less likely to be compressed within these structures, but can be irritated and traumatised following atrophy (thinning) of the heel fat pad (Kopell and Thompson, 1960; Davidson and Copoloff, 1990). Pain is usually felt more towards the back of the heel.

Entrapment of the Medial Plantar Nerve

Entrapment of the MPN is not as common as entrapment of the other nerves (Murphy and Baxter 1985), particularly as an isolated entity (Raikin and Schon 2000). Out of 21 cases diagnosed with nerve entrapment in the ankle and foot, Murphy and Baxter (1985) concluded that only one case was consistent with MPN entrapment (cited in Alshami et al 2008).

Entrapment of the Tibial Nerve (Tarsal Tunnel Syndrome)

Tarsal tunnel syndrome is a more common condition of the foot and ankle than has been historically appreciated. It is a compression or entrapment of the tibial nerve which is a branch of the large sciatic nerve. It runs across the inside of the ankle joint, just behind the ankle bone (the tarsal tunnel). At this point, the nerve splits into smaller branches which run into the heel and the sole of the foot. Compression of this nerve may cause radiating pain into the heel and further along the foot into the toes. Currently, it is a condition that is largely under-diagnosed as a potential cause of heel pain, arch pain, and distal peripheral neuropathy. False-negative electrodiagnostic testing contributes to the under-diagnosis of tarsal tunnel syndrome. This is where the diagnostic test does not pick up any abnormalities in the nerve and muscle firing patterns however these tests are not 100% accurate and therefore can miss a problem with the nerve. It is also reported to be the most common chronic nerve entrapment in the lower extremity (Dellon 1996).

What causes tarsal tunnel syndrome?

It is most often believed to be caused by "space-occupying lesions," such as soft tissue or bony lumps and bumps within the tarsal tunnel that shouldn't be there. Examples include ganglia or lipoma (fatty tissue mass), varicosities such as varicose veins which increase pressure on the nerve, fibrosis (thickening) of the tibial nerve itself which may have been triggered by injury. Other proposed causes include biomechanical issues such as collapse feet or excessively high arched feet as both these extremes narrow the space in the tarsal tunnel and may lead to compression of the nerve.

Presentation of neural pain

Heel pain of neural origin typically presents as a burning, sharp, shooting, electrical pain with pins and needles, numbness. Pain is worse during weight-bearing and relieved by rest. However, pain may also be present during non-weight bearing. It has been suggested that pain at night may be due to nerve compression as a result of venostasis (slowing of venous outflow) and venous engorgement which results in increased compression of the soft tissues of the foot and ankle (Kopell & Thompson 1960; Doxey, 1987). Like plantar fasciitis, it is very common to experience pain first thing in the morning and after long periods of rest.

So how do I know if it's plantar fasciitis or neural heel pain?

This is not an easy question to answer even for competent, experienced clinicians. This is why it is a very challenging problem for both patients and clinicians. The fact that the conservative management of plantar heel pain is still challenging can be attributed to the difficulties in establishing the correct differential diagnosis and cause.

It is recommended that you see a podiatrist or suitable specialist to perform a clinical examination to help achieve the right diagnosis before considering diagnostic testing

Diagnostic Testing

There are various diagnostic tests to help confirm neurogenic pain whether it be from compression of one of the small plantar nerves of the heel or the tibial nerve. It is important to point out that diagnostic testing should complement the physical examination and should not be relied upon to make an accurate diagnosis.

MRI

An MRI can be ordered to help confirm a diagnosis. MRI may also be useful in establishing the presence of a space-occupying lesion beneath the flexor retinaculum at the ankle joint resulting in tarsal tunnel syndrome, which can mimic symptoms of plantar fasciitis. However, the incidence of such lesions is rare. Some studies have reported MRI to be highly accurate (82%–83%) in the diagnosis of tarsal tunnel syndrome (Reade et al 2001).

Diagnostic Ultrasound

Diagnostic ultrasound is less frequently ordered when suspicious of nerve entrapment and currently there is no evidence to support its accuracy. But it can be used to check for synovitis of peripheral tendon sheaths such as the posterior tibial and flexor tendons about the ankle. Ganglia and space- occupying lesions can also be identified in the region of the tarsal tunnel or surrounding structures.

The tibial nerve and its branches can also be traced to evaluate the potential presence of a high division; this can result in overfill of the tarsal canal by the medial and lateral plantar nerve branches. Tests are often performed using a high-frequency type machine

Electrodiagnostic Studies

Electrodiagnostic studies have traditionally been the gold standard for confirming and evaluating the clinical diagnosis of tarsal tunnel syndrome. Motor and sensory nerve conduction studies (NCS) and electromyography (EMG) should be evaluated. EMG may show motor latencies in the abductor hallucis (muscle connected to the big toe) or abductor digiti minimi (muscle connected to the little toe). It has been suggested that sensory action potentials are a more sensitive test. False negative NCS and EMG are not uncommon, and so, unfortunately, do not rule out tarsal tunnel syndrome (Franson & Baravarian 2006).

Quantitative Sensory Testing

A more recent diagnostic tool is computer-assisted quantitative sensory testing, also known as a pressure-specified sensory device or PSSD (Dellon 1996). This neurosensory testing device has been shown to provide a more sensitive appreciation of peripheral nerve compromise, which can confirm a clinical diagnosis earlier in the progression of tarsal tunnel syndrome. The PSSD machine is designed to address the subtle changes that occur in peripheral nerves as nerve damage increases.

Treatment

If you have seen a podiatrist or suitably qualified specialist who suspects neural heel pain then you have probably been advised on the general non-surgical treatments used to treat plantar fasciitis including rest, anti-inflammatories, night splint, foot orthoses (insoles) to correct any biomechanical abnormalities, soft soled shoes, foot supports, massage roller, stretching exercises for the Achilles tendon and plantar fascia, extra-corporeal shockwave therapy, corticosteroid injections, cast immobilisation etc. Surprisingly the treatment plan for heel pain whether it is plantar fasciitis or neural heel pain is almost identical.

Additional non-surgical treatment one should try if neural heel pain is suspected is neural mobilisation techniques. To find out more about these please visit our the links below:

https://www.youtube.com/edit?o=U&video_id=qX7QwSTD-bE

https://www.youtube.com/edit?o=U&video_id=mJWNKhLT0Sk

https://www.youtube.com/edit?o=U&video_id=IJ2nWh3YS9k

Surgical management

Surgery is considered if conservative treatment has failed usually at least after 12 months. There are many surgical procedures for treating heel pain and often a combination of procedures are performed during the surgery. With regards to isolated procedures involving a surgical release of the offending nerve previous studies have reported excellent outcomes with 83% of patients reporting complete resolution of pain involving 69 heels (Baxter & Pfeffer 1992). A study by Hendrix and colleagues (1998) reported 90% complete resolution in symptoms following surgical decompression of tarsal tunnel which relieves the tibial nerve.

Generally, surgical release of nerve entrapment has a good post-op recovery as it involves minimal damage to the surrounding soft tissue of the foot and ankle and usually no damage to bone unless there is a bony problem causing the entrapment. If neurogenic heel pain has not responded to non-surgical treatment, then surgical release should be considered as a suitable treatment option.

Summary

Heel pain of neural origin is often overlooked. Proper patient education about this condition is of paramount importance in order to help patients self-manage and improve their pain. Clinicians should suspect a neural component to a patient's pain if symptoms aren't improving as expected and consider diagnostic tests to help get to the route of the problem. Once this is achieved then the most appropriate management plan can be put in place.

Inflammatory Disease and Heel Pain

When plantar fasciitis does not respond as expected to conservative treatment one should always consider other potential causes of heel pain including underlying inflammatory disease.

There are many different types of inflammatory diseases and this section will review some of the more common inflammatory conditions which are linked to heel pain.

Blood Tests

The initial workup for an inflammatory cause of heel pain should start with basic blood tests. Blood tests allow the investigator to assess whether you may have abnormal levels of specific blood characteristics. Common characteristics involved in inflammatory disease include rheumatoid factor (RF), human leukocyte antigen 27 (HLA-B27), antinuclear antigen (ANA), erythrocyte sedimentation rate (ESR) and c-reactive protein (CRP). Certain inflammatory diseases have strong associations with certain blood characteristics. This information helps the clinician to make an accurate diagnosis and help the patient understand why they have heel pain.

Rheumatoid factor (RF) - Rheumatoid factor is an antibody that is measurable in the blood. Rheumatoid factor is actually an antibody that can bind to other antibodies. Antibodies are normal proteins in our blood that are important parts of our immune system. Rheumatoid factor is an antibody that is not usually present in the normal individual and can be positive in 75% to 85% of rheumatoid patients, therefore it is a very insightful test when investigating a possible inflammatory disease.

Human leukocyte antigen B27 (HLA-B27) - Human leukocyte antigen B27 (HLA-B27) is a blood test that identifies a specific protein located on the surface of your white blood cells called human leukocyte antigen B27. Human leukocyte antigens (HLAs) are proteins commonly found on white blood cells. These antigens help your immune system identify differences between healthy body tissue and foreign substances that may cause infection. Although most HLAs protect the body from harm, HLA-B27 is a specific type of protein that contributes to immune system dysfunction.

The presence of HLA-B27 on your white blood cells can cause your immune system to attack the healthy cells that contain it. HLA-B27 has a sensitivity of approximately 90% to 95% in ankylosing spondylitis, 80% in Reiter syndrome, 50% in inflammatory bowel disease, and 70% in psoriasis.

Antinuclear antigen (ANA) - Antibodies develop in your immune system to help the body fight infectious organisms. When an antibody recognizes the foreign proteins of an infectious organism, it recruits other proteins and cells to fight off the infection. This cascade of attack is called inflammation. Unfortunately, some antibodies make incorrect calls, identifying a naturally-occurring protein as foreign. These autoantibodies start the cascade of inflammation, causing the body to attack itself. Most of us have autoantibodies, but typically in small amounts. The presence of a lot of autoantibodies or ANAs can indicate an autoimmune disease. ANA is positive in 95% of patients with systemic lupus erythematosus (SLE), but it can be seen in patients with rheumatoid arthritis and Sjogren's syndrome.

Erythrocyte sedimentation rate (ESR) - ESR measures the rate at which the red blood cells separate from the plasma and fall to the bottom of a test tube. If certain proteins cover red cells, these will stick to each other and cause the red cells to fall more quickly. A high ESR indicates that you have some inflammation, somewhere in the body.

C-reactive protein (CRP) - CRP is produced by the liver. The level of CRP rises when there is inflammation throughout the body. The CRP test is a general test to check for inflammation in the body. It is not a specific test. That means it can reveal that you have inflammation somewhere in your body, but it cannot pinpoint the exact location.

Both ESR and CRP tests are nonspecific and can be used to

monitor the progression of an inflammatory process.

Anticyclic citrullinated peptide antibody (Anti CCP antibody) - Anti CCP antibodies are autoantibodies, meaning they are antibodies directed against an individual's own proteins. they are present in the majority of patients with rheumatoid arthritis.

Rheumatoid Arthritis

Diagnosis of rheumatoid arthritis is based on criteria set by the American College of Rheumatology (Arnett 1988)

1) Morning stiffness greater than 1 hour
2) Arthritis of 3 or more joint areas; right or left finger and toe joints, metacarpophalangeal joint (Hand), wrist, elbow, knee, ankle, and metatarsal phalangeal joint (balls of foot)
3) Arthritis of hand joints (swelling in at least 1 area: Wrist, PIPJ, or MCPJ)
4) Symmetric arthritis
5) Rheumatoid nodules
6) Serum RF (Rheumatoid factor positive in blood test)
7) X-ray changes.

The first 4 criteria must have been present for at least 6 weeks. 4 out of 7 criteria must be present for the diagnosis of rheumatoid arthritis.

The onset of rheumatoid arthritis is between the third and fifth decade of life. The prevalence is approximately 0.8% of the world population with women affected 2 to 2.5 times more than men. RF is present in about 75% to 85% of patients with rheumatoid arthritis. Anti-CCP and RF can present 10 years before the onset of symptoms and can be useful in starting preventative treatment.

RA and Heel Pain

Radiographic findings particular to the calcaneus (heel bone) in rheumatoid arthritis include erosion of the bone and above the insertion of the Achilles tendon. Heel spurs are also commonly seen (Resnick et al 1977). The reason for the development of plantar heel pain in rheumatoid arthritis is largely unknown. A study by Falsetti and colleagues in 2004 revealed the presence of a pattern of inflammation and oedema of the heel pad in 6.6% of patients with rheumatoid arthritis. Their ultrasound based study revealed the possibility that there is focal rupture of the fibrous septae of the heel pad along with necrosis of the fat pad. Most of the patients with this observed pattern had associated heel pain.

Treatment of rheumatoid arthritis centres on early diagnosis. The more the disease has progressed, the worse the prognosis. Once the disease is diagnosed, treatment needs to be aggressive to prevent joint destruction. The patient should be referred to a rheumatologist. Nonsteroidal anti-inflammatory drugs (NSAIDs), disease-modifying antirheumatic drugs (DMARDs) and corticosteroids are used depending on the severity of the disease. Physical and occupational therapy should be instituted to retain joint function.

Ankylosing Spondylitis

Ankylosing spondylitis mainly affects the spine and sacroiliac joint (part of the pelvis). Sacroiliitis is the first recognized clinical symptom of the disease. The onset is in late adolescent or early adulthood and it is rarely seen to develop after the age of 40 years. Men are twice as likely to develop the disease as women. Its worldwide prevalence can range from 0.1% to 6%.

The disease initially presents as back pain in the gluteus or sacroiliac joint region. Clinical features of ankylosing spondylitis include inflammation and arthritis of the hips and shoulders, peripheral arthritis, enthesitis, osteoporosis, spinal fracture, pseudoarthrosis, acute inflammation of the eyes, and heart. The primary clinical feature is a loss of spinal mobility.

The clinical diagnosis of ankylosing spondylitis is made based on the 1984 modified New York Criteria:

X-ray findings

Clinical findings including:

- Low-back pain and stiffness greater than 3 months that improves with exercise but not rest
- Limitation of motion of the lumbar spine (lower back) when bending frontwards and sideways
- Limitation of chest expansion compared with normal values for age and sex.

The condition is definitely ankylosing spondylitis if the x-ray finding is associated with at least 1 clinical criterion.

AS and Heel Pain

Enthesitis of ankylosing spondylitis, which is inflammation of the attachment points of ligaments and capsule (Bluestone 1982) can lead to Achilles tendonitis and plantar fasciitis. Posterior and plantar heel pain can present clinically, differentiating ankylosing spondylitis from typical heel pain. Insertional Achilles tendinopathy is commonly accompanied by bursitis. X-rays can reveal the presence of a fluffy periosteal (bone) reaction at this site. In addition, the following x-ray findings may be seen: erosion of the back aspect of the heel above the Achilles tendon insertion, heel spur at the site of insertion of the Achilles tendon, and erosion of the bottom aspect of the heel distal to the origin of the plantar fascia (Resnick et al 1977).

However, the most common x-ray findings are seen in the pelvis. Osteitis and osseous erosion are features of the disease at points of ligamentous or tendinous attachment. Continuation of the disease process leads to the replacement of local tissues with fibrocartilage that will eventually ossify. This process is seen with the development of a bamboo spine.

HLA-B27 (mentioned in blood tests earlier) is seen in more than 90% of patients with ankylosing spondylitis and has a sensitivity of approximately 95%. Increased CRP and ESR are seen in 50% to 75% of patients with ankylosing spondylitis.

Ankylosing spondylitis predominately affects the ankle and heel rather than the balls of the feet. The lack of abnormal skin features distinguishes this disease from other seronegative arthropathies. Treatment of ankylosing spondylitis consists of early diagnosis, NSAIDs, and daily exercises.

Psoriatic Arthritis and Heel Pain

Psoriatic arthritis affects up to one in five people with psoriasis (a common skin condition). Often the presenting heel pain will be unilateral (only in one foot). Skin presentations include silvery scaled, red plaques along tops of the feet surfaces and nail changes including pitting, and brown-yellow discoloration, also known as the oil drop sign. Nail changes are predictive of those patients who will develop psoriatic arthritis.

X-rays show erosion of the back the calcaneus (heel bone) above the Achilles tendon insertion, with spurring at the site of insertion of the Achilles tendon, plantar heel spur at the origin of the plantar fascia, and erosion of the plantar aspect of the calcaneus distal to the origin of the plantar fascia (Resnick 1977). Enthesitis is a common feature of the disease and can cause heel pain through inflammation of the insertion of the Achilles tendon and origin of the plantar fascia. An effusion of the retrocalcaneal bursa is also often present. These x-ray features distinguish from typical heel pain and can identify an undiagnosed inflammatory disease.

Treatment of disease is focused on controlling the inflammation with NSAIDs, disease modifying drugs (DMARDs) and sometimes biologic drugs. The heel pain can be treated with NSAIDs, injections to control inflammation along with physical therapy including stretching exercises, footwear, orthoses and shockwave therapy.

Reiter Syndrome and Heel Pain

Reiter syndrome is a form reactive arthritis caused by exposure to infectious disease with Chlamydia being the most common infection. Over 60% of patients with Reiter syndrome suffer from heel pain. Like other inflammatory conditions Reiter syndrome also causes abnormal changes seen on x-rays at the heel bone which help distinguish it from typical heel pain. An irregular plantar heel spur due to erosion and bone formation at the origin of the plantar fascia will commonly be noted

Reiter syndrome is a self-limiting disease that usually resolves within a year. However, some patients will continue to have chronic (long term) musculoskeletal problems. Chronic foot pain specifically in the joints of the rearfoot and heel pain is the major clinical symptoms.

Sarcoidosis and Heel Pain

Sarcoidosis is more prevalent in the African American population than in the White population. The disease process presents between 20 and 40 years of age. It is a granulomatous disease. Chronic granulomatous disease is an inherited disorder in which immune system cells called phagocytes do not function properly. This leads to ongoing and severe infection. It can affect all organ systems and can produce rheumatic manifestations in 10% to 15% of patients. It has been reported that practically all patients with sarcoidosis suffer from heel pain in the early stage. Shaw and colleagues reported that all of the patients in their study had heel pain during the acute stage of the disease.

Gout and Heel Pain

Gout usually presents clinically in joints. This disease process is due to the overproduction or under secretion of uric acid. Uric acid crystals are needle-shaped. The big toe of the foot is the most commonly affected site in the foot. Radiographically, bone erosions, described as rat-bite lesions, of the first metatarsal head are commonly seen. Heel pain can manifest secondary to the presence of tophus deposits about the heel bone, specifically about the Achilles tendon and its insertion and less commonly at the plantar heel. For symptomatic tophus deposits, surgical excision may be indicated (Lichniak 1990). Treatment is aimed at controlling inflammation and lowering a person's uric acid levels.

Summary

The clinical course of heel pain can be frustrating to the clinician and the patient. Most heel pain responds to conservative care in a short period of time. However, when heel pain is resistant to treatment, other causes should be considered. A detailed history and physical examination, along with appropriate laboratory tests including blood tests and diagnostic studies, can direct the clinician toward the correct diagnosis. There are many inflammatory causes of heel pain, some common and others uncommon. Regardless of the incidence, a strong index of suspicion is raised whenever the heel pain fails to respond as routine plantar fasciitis should.

Heel pain and Hyperparathyroidism

When plantar fasciitis does not respond as expected to conservative treatment one should always consider other potential causes of heel pain. Hyperparathyroidism is a metabolic disorder in which parathyroid hormone is secreted in excess. This overproduction of the hormone results in osteoporosis (brittle bone disease). Clinical signs of hyperparathyroidism include hypercalcemia (high levels of calcium in the blood), recurrent kidney stones, mental status changes, fatigue, depression, gastrointestinal distress, and back pain.

How is hyperparathyroidism diagnosed?

Hyperparathyroidism is usually diagnosed after blood tests have shown a high level of calcium and a high level of parathyroid hormone. Usually, the level of phosphate in your blood is low.

If you have secondary hyperparathyroidism, your blood calcium level may be low or normal but you will still have a raised parathyroid hormone level. If you also have kidney disease, your blood phosphate level can be high because your kidney cannot get rid of (excrete) phosphate in your urine.

Heel Pain Case

Fishco and colleagues (1999) presented a case of chronic heel pain initially diagnosed as plantar fasciitis that failed to respond to usual treatment. On presentation, the patient had a medical history significant for multiple spinal fractures, recurrent kidney stones, and gastrointestinal disease. The patient was later diagnosed with a stress fracture of the heel bone secondary to hyperparathyroidism. The patient's calcium levels in her blood were normal but her parathyroid hormone was greatly increased. An iliac crest bone biopsy confirmed the diagnosis.

Heel pain and Sickle Cell Anaemia

What is sickle cell anaemia?

Sickle cell anaemia is a serious inherited blood disorder where the red blood cells, which carry oxygen around the body, develop abnormally. The disorder mainly affects people of African, Caribbean, Middle Eastern, Eastern Mediterranean and Asian origin. In the UK, sickle cell disorders are most commonly seen in African and Caribbean people.

How is it diagnosed?

Sickle cell anaemia can be diagnosed using a blood test to check for defective haemoglobin. A small amount of defective haemoglobin would suggest that you have the sickle cell trait (you're a carrier of the sickle cell gene), but don't have sickle cell anaemia. A high level of defective haemoglobin would indicate that you have sickle cell anaemia.

Heel Pain

Sickle cell anaemia causes clotting of the microvascular circulation (small blood vessels) supplying bones, which results in aseptic necrosis. Aseptic necrosis is the death of body tissue due to poor blood supply. Aseptic necrosis of the heel bone has been reported in the literature but is rare. Radiographic findings include patchy sclerosis, cortical thickening, and osteopaenia. Rothschild & Sebes (1981) conducted a study that evaluated 100 patients with sickle cell anaemia. They discovered erosions of the posterior superior aspect of the heel bone in 14% of their patients and believed this to be linked to sickle cell anaemia. However, this area of the heel pain is not in the location of the plantar fascia thus sickle cell anaemia may have a poor causal link with plantar fasciitis related heel pain but may help explain pain at the back of the heel which hasn't responded to usual treatments.

Plantar Fibromatosis

Plantar fibromatosis is a benign (non-cancerous) soft tissue tumour located at the bottom of the foot usually on top of the plantar fascia along the arch of the foot. It is also known as Lederhose disease.

Due to the location of this tumour, it may be confused with plantar fasciitis. These tumours vary in size and many are nonpainful for a long time, often until they grow large, protruding prominently under the skin. It is reported that the average size of is approximately 1.1cm and mostly demonstrates an elongated shape as opposed to a round or oval shape (Bedi & Davidson 2001). Plantar fibromatosis can often be diagnosed clinically however diagnostic imaging such as ultrasound or MRI can be helpful to confirm a diagnosis in less obvious cases (if the tumour is too small to see in a clinical setting). Diagnostic ultrasound is recommended as the imaging modality of choice due to its cost effectiveness over MRI (Bedi & Davidson 2001).

Treatment

Not all cases of plantar fibromatosis require treatment as some cases are nonpainful and can spontaneously resolve however in painful cases the most effective treatment is to offload pressure from the lesion. Pain is produced on weight bearing such as standing and walking. Most patient's respond very well to an offloading device such as an orthosis (insole) with a deflective pad to reduce compression of the fibroma. Rarely do these lesions need to be excised (surgically removed). A small number of cases may require surgical removal, however, surgery is not without its complications. Patients may be left with painful scarring after surgical removal due to the scar line being on the bottom of the foot which can become aggravated when walking. In some cases, the fibroma tissue is embedded within the plantar fascia and foot muscles. This makes removal more difficult and can lead to damage and weakening of the plantar fascia and plantar foot muscles which can lead to secondary problems. There is also a high recurrence rate following surgical excision.

Summary

Plantar fibromatosis is a benign soft tissue mass that is often visible clinically, however in cases of smaller plantar fibroma's that may not be seen clinically, this condition may be confused with plantar fasciitis due to the location of the tumour (on top of or within the plantar fascia). The symptom pattern of painful plantar fibromatosis may be confused with plantar fasciitis as both conditions are exacerbated by weight-bearing and relieved by rest. When suspected plantar fasciitis is not responding to usual treatment one should always consider diagnostic testing such as ultrasound which can assess the plantar fascia for thickening which confirms plantar fasciitis. In the absence of plantar fascia thickening, the sonographer may look for other abnormalities such as a hypoechoic mass which is indicative of a plantar fibroma. Most plantar fibroma's respond well to simple offloading with an orthosis and surgical excision should not be taken lightly for this condition.

Plantar Fascia Rupture

Plantar fascia rupture was first reported by Leach in 1978. Since then it has not been reported frequently which may due to the condition being rare or that it is often not recognised. It is believed that plantar fascia tear is rare because the plantar fascia is thick, tough, and resilient to pressure and trauma (Healey & Chen 2010).

The patient history is very important in helping accurately diagnose a plantar fascia rupture. Patients present with a history of trauma, a feeling of sharp pain, often accompanied by a pop or a tearing sensation in the plantar heel or arch area. The presentation includes swelling and often bruising. A palpable defect in the fascia may be present. Confirmation by MRI or ultrasound may be necessary, although plantar fascia tear is often a clinical diagnosis.

The mechanism of injury is an acceleration type of motion that typically precedes the painful event in which the fascia ruptures such as pushing off at the toes during walking or running. Chronic repetitive stress and minor repetitive trauma contribute to the development of the tears which can lead to a rupture (Christman 2003). Plantar fascia rupture has also been correlated with previous multiple corticosteroid injections to the plantar fascia (Acvedo & Besin 1998). Treatment includes immobilisation, rest, ice, NSAIDs, and non–weight bearing with crutches, often for a period of 4 to 6 weeks. Following this patient's should make a very gradual return to normal activities wearing a supportive shoe and foot orthoses to provide maximum protection of the foot for short to midterm use.

Chapter Six

Diagnostic Modalities for Heel Pain

Diagnostic imaging modalities come in many forms, with each possessing strengths and limitations in their usefulness for diagnosing chronic heel pain that has failed to respond to treatment. This section will review the main diagnostic imaging modalities used to help diagnose heel pain.

X-rays

X-rays have been, and are still, the most commonly used imaging tool used to help diagnose heel pain. The most common cause of heel pain by far is plantar fasciitis. X-rays, however, assess for bony abnormality and do not provide information on the soft tissues. As plantar fasciitis is a soft tissue condition an x-ray cannot be used to confirm a diagnosis of plantar fasciitis which begs the question why are x-rays the most common imaging tool for heel pain? The answer is that plantar fasciitis is diagnosed clinically through a detailed patient history and physical examination. Patients should not be referred for x-rays to confirm plantar fasciitis but instead to investigate for other causes of heel pain such as bony abnormalities. However, more times than not the x-ray findings are reported as normal. Occasionally the x-ray finding may identify a heel spur but currently, there is no evidence to prove a causal relationship between heel spurs and plantar fasciitis. Furthermore, there is evidence against a causal link between plantar heel spurs and plantar fasciitis which comes from anatomical and MRI studies (for more information on this see chapter 11). Despite this x-rays do have their use and can also confirm later-stage stress fractures, bone tumours, bone cysts, periostitis, and erosions due to infection or rheumatologic causes.

Diagnostic Ultrasound

Diagnostic ultrasound is considered the imaging modality of choice. Unlike x-ray which looks for other causes of heel pain, ultrasound can be used to confirm the diagnosis of plantar fasciitis as it investigates the health and appearance of the plantar fascia. In patients with clinical symptoms of plantar fasciitis, the proximal end of the fascia is hypoechoic, which can be seen clearly when compared with the surrounding soft tissue. The plantar fascia is also significantly thicker in patients with plantar fasciitis. Symptomatic patients were seen to have fascia measuring more than 4mm in thickness, whereas those of asymptomatic patients measured 4 mm or less. A potential limitation with diagnostic ultrasound is that it is operator-dependent meaning the accuracy of the test relies heavily on the skills and experience of the person operating the machine.

Ultrasound has been useful in the diagnosis of other causes of heel pain. For example, a retrocalcaneal bursa is seen as fluid between the Achilles tendon and the calcaneus (heel bone). A retro-Achilles bursa is fluid lying deep to the tendon. Fat pad atrophy (thinning of the fat pad) is demonstrated by discrete fluid between fat lobules in the plantar aspect of the foot with thinning of the fat. Upon compression, this gets even thinner and is much more compliant than the normal plantar fat. Colour Doppler is useful in diagnosing plantar vein thrombosis. Doppler flow is not generally seen, except for in association with perifascial fluid, in discrete distal nodules and at the calcaneal origin when there are erosions. This latter appearance is very rare and is seen as an extension of Achilles insertional change and erosions, presumably secondary to inflammatory disease (Ieong et al 2013). Colour Doppler can also be used to assess for the presence of neovascularisation which is an influx of intra-fascia arterial blood supply. This is believed to contribute to the pathological process and increased hypersensitivity of the tissue, however, there are conflicting views on the significance of this finding among the medical profession.

MRI

Similar to x-rays, MRI is more useful to rule out other causes of heel pain than to confirm a diagnosis of plantar fasciitis, such as tarsal tunnel syndrome, ganglion, infection or tumour. Usual MRI findings include thickening of the plantar fascia, swelling around the plantar fascia, bone marrow oedema of the heel, stress fracture, and tearing of the plantar fascia. A benefit from MRI over x-rays is that it can identify both soft tissue and bony tissue abnormalities and provides richer information which is more useful when investigating the cause of chronic heel pain. MRI may also be useful in establishing the presence of a space-occupying lesion beneath the flexor retinaculum at the ankle joint resulting in tarsal tunnel syndrome, which can mimic symptoms of plantar fasciitis. However, the incidence of such lesions is rare, and it would be hard to justify the expense of this test unless the examiner's index of suspicion was extremely high for such pathology.

Computerized Tomography (CT) Scan

Computerized tomography (CT) scans are generally only considered in cases of nonrespondent heel pain and if other causes of heel pain are suspected such as calcaneal stress fracture.

Technetium 99 Bone Scan

A bone scan is often positive with chronic heel pain and plantar fasciitis due to chronic periostitis and inflammation, with increased activity in the periosteum. A technetium 99 bone scan can also diagnose fatigue or a stress fracture. There will be diffuse, intense increased activity with a stress fracture, whereas plantar fasciitis will show focal uptake in the area of the medial calcaneal tuberosity. This imaging modality seems to be mentioned in textbooks however I have never personally referred a patient for this type of scan and I don't know a single colleague that has either. I think the reason for this is that other options have demonstrated superiority over this method and it has never become outdated.

Electrodiagnostic study - Nerve Conduction Velocity and Electromyography Test

A complete electrodiagnostic study involves nerve conduction studies (NCS) and electromyography (EMG). The two complement each other, in that both give information about peripheral nerves and muscles. Each in isolation does not yield a complete assessment of the cause of the symptoms being assessed in a limb or limbs.

In the first portion of the electrodiagnostic study, nerve conduction velocity test is used to measure the function of the nerves in the body. This test is performed if tarsal tunnel nerve entrapment is suspected. Normal scores are 4.1 and 4.7 milliseconds for the medial and lateral plantar nerves, respectively. Patients with tarsal tunnel syndrome show delays in the nerve conduction velocity studies. However, in some cases of tarsal tunnel, these studies may be normal. In the second portion of the electrodiagnostic study, needle electromyography, a narrow needle electrode is inserted into the belly of the muscle being investigated while the patient voluntarily contracts the muscle.

Although some literature suggests that only the presence of delayed nerve conduction velocity can establish the diagnosis of neurogenic heel pain, other authors believe that the diagnosis is a clinical one to make.

Electrodiagnostic studies have traditionally been the gold standard for confirming and evaluating the clinical diagnosis of tarsal tunnel syndrome. However false negative NCS and EMG are not uncommon, and so, unfortunately, do not rule out tarsal tunnel syndrome.

Pressure-specific sensory testing

A more recent diagnostic tool is computer-assisted quantitative sensory testing, also known as a pressure-specified sensory device or PSSD (Dellon 1996). This neurosensory testing device has been shown to provide a more sensitive appreciation of peripheral nerve compromise, which can confirm a clinical diagnosis earlier in the progression of tarsal tunnel syndrome. The PSSD machine is designed to address the subtle changes that occur in peripheral nerves as nerve damage increases. PSSD may also be of benefit in evaluating the effects of surgical releases, but it should not be regarded as a replacement for a thorough history and physical examination.

Choosing the right test

There is no one perfect modality for diagnosing chronic heel pain that is superior to other tests. Each test comes with its unique benefits and limitations. The traditional practice of referring patients for an x-ray as a first line diagnostic test should be challenged as this rarely provides further insight to the diagnosis. Instead, the diagnostic modality choice should be guided by a thorough patient history and physical examination by a competent clinician. This will allow the clinician to choose the most appropriate test(s) relevant to the individual patient.

Chapter Seven

Soft Tissue Stress & Injury to the Plantar Fascia

Physiological Stress (normal injury free stress)

When bodily tissue is subjected to an external loading force it will develop an internal resistance to that load, which is called stress. The body's musculoskeletal system (soft tissue and bones) is designed to withstand continuous stress on a daily basis. Stress on these structures is a perfectly natural process of living. In fact, if stress levels are completely eliminated on a specific body part this can lead to atrophy (wastage of tissue) which can have a negative effect on daily living. An example of this would be the effects on the calf muscle following long-term immobilisation in a below knee cast. As the amount of force being applied to the calf muscle is considerably reduced this causes atrophy of the calf muscle. Muscle atrophy will hinder normal muscle function to perform simple activities such as walking. This is why rehabilitation is often required for patients who have had long term cast immobilisation in order to re-develop muscle strength.

The external forces that cause stresses to occur within a structure may be classified by the way they tend to deform the structure upon which they are acting. These forces can be broken down into 3 main types

- Compressive stress
- Tensile Stress
- Shear stress

Compressive Stress

Compressive stress occurs when the structure develops an internal loading force that tends to make it resist being pushed together, for instance, the tibia (shin bone) develops compressive stress in response to supporting the mass of the body during weight bearing activities.

Tensile Stress

Tensile stress occurs when the structure develops an internal loading force that to resist being pulled apart, for instance, the plantar fascia develops tensile stress in response to arch lowering in the foot.

Shear Stress

Any forces acting parallel, or tangential, to the applied external loading force creates a shear stress. Shear stress is commonly developed in structures where torsional forces are applied to that structure.

Pathological Stress (excessive stress and injury)

When a material is elastic, it will deform a certain amount upon application of an external loading force and then will return to its original shape once the loading force has been removed. However, at higher loading forces, a material will undergo permanent or plastic deformation, which will cause the material to permanently change shape, fracture or rupture (Ozkaya & Nihat 1999). Stress levels can be described by using a stress-strain curve. This is a common concept in engineering. You can Google this term to find plenty of images on this.

In order to remain injury free, the structural materials of an individual's body (i.e bone, cartilage, skin, fascia, tendon and ligament must function at stress levels that are within the elastic region of its stress-strain curve. In this way when a loading force is applied to that material, the material will deform temporarily in response to that loading force and then return to its original size and shape once the loading force is removed. For example, if a bone is loaded by a compression force, it will shorten slightly in response to that force and then, once compression force is removed, will lengthen back to its original shape. In addition, if a ligament or tendon is loaded by a tension force, it will lengthen in response to that force and then shorten back to its original length when the tension force is removed. However, if bone, cartilage, skin, muscle, tendon, fascia or ligament is loaded above its elastic limit, then plastic deformation of that biologic material will occur. For example, excessive compression loads on a bone may cause a compression fracture and excessive tensile loads on a tendon or ligament may cause a lengthening, partial rupture or complete rupture of that structure. Therefore when body tissue is within its elastic region this can be deemed physiological stress and when a body tissue is beyond this point and undergoes plastic deformation this can be deemed pathological stress which leads to injury and potential rupture.

In plantar fasciitis it is believed that the plantar fascia undergoes pathological tensile stress, resulting in micro-tearing of the fascia which leads to tissue degeneration if not resolved.

Chapter Eight

Biomechanical Theory of Plantar Fasciitis

It is commonly believed that plantar fasciitis is caused by excess mechanical stress, with the main type of stress being tensile stress within the plantar fascia (described in chapter seven). However, the plantar fascia is also subject to high levels of compressive stress that are generated as the heel strikes the ground. Therefore the plantar fascia is subjected to high levels of both tensile stress and compressive stress during weight bearing activities, either or both of which may be responsible for painful plantar fasciitis symptoms. Furthermore the repetitive nature of walking results in repetitive loading and unloading of both tensile stress and compressive stress within the plantar fascia with each step. This leads to a situation where there is a repetitive injury to the plantar fascia that delays or prevents healing from occurring (Kirby 2009). Thus it is highly possible that it is this combination of high levels of both tensile and compressive stress on the plantar fascia that makes plantar fasciitis such a common problem in society today.

The Windlass Mechanism

The Windlass Mechanism is a crucial component of normal foot function. A disruption to the windlass mechanism is believed to result in abnormal foot function which can lead to a wide range of biomechanical issues. The windlass mechanism was first described by Hicks in 1954. It is a mechanical model that provides a detailed explanation of the biomechanical factors and stresses placed on the plantar fascia during normal human function. Hicks described the foot and its ligaments as an arch-like triangular structure or truss. The heel, midtarsal joint, and metatarsals (the arch of the foot) form the truss' arch. The plantar fascia forms the tie-rod that runs from the heel to the toes. Vertical forces from body weight travel downward via the tibia (shin bone) and tend to flatten the arch. Furthermore, ground reaction forces travel upward on the heel and the balls of the feet, which can further attenuate the flattening effect (Bolgla & Malone 2004).

A triangle can be drawn to demonstrate the truss formed by the heel bone, midtarsal joint, and metatarsals. The hypotenuse (horizontal line) represents the plantar fascia. The upward arrows depict ground reaction forces. The downward arrow depicts the body's vertical force. The orientation of the vertical and ground reaction forces would cause a collapse of the truss; however, increased plantar fascia tension in response to these forces maintains the truss' integrity.

Dysfunctional Windlass Mechanism

Since the windlass mechanism is considered crucial for normal foot function, dysfunction of the windlass mechanism results in abnormal function and thus increased stress placed on the lower limb structures, namely the plantar fascia. One reason why the windlass mechanism may become disrupted is limited dorsiflexion (upwards flexion) of the big toe during walking. It is commonly reported that increased foot pronation results in limited dorsiflexion of the big toe joint. It is also commonly reported that tight calf muscles are one of the leading forces contributing to increased foot pronation. Therefore in a person with tight calf muscles, the foot may be undergo increased foot pronation which may block or limit dorsiflexion of the big toe joint. To overcome this limited dorsiflexion of the big toe joint, the plantar fascia is placed under increased stress, since more force is needed to dorsiflex the big toe and activate the windlass mechanism. This increased repetitive stress results in micro tearing and strain in the plantar fascia which leads to plantar fasciitis.

Restoring the Windlass Mechanism

The aim of biomechanical treatment is to influence biomechanical function and optimise the windlass mechanism. The main way of achieving this goal is via foot orthoses, usually designed to control foot pronation. We do not know how exactly foot orthoses work, however by using biomechanical theoretical models we can infer that foot orthoses will increase the supination moment acting on the foot thus decreasing pronation moment. A decrease in pronation moment may restore the windlass mechanism, allowing the plantar fascia to function in a state of physiological stress leading to tissue healing and resolution of pain.

Chapter Nine

Miscellaneous Topics

Plantar Fasciitis or Heel Spur? The Chicken or The Egg?

Patients often ask "*Do I have a heel spur or do I have plantar fasciitis?*"

This is a conundrum which comes up time and time again and is possibly due to the two terms being used synonymously by different healthcare professionals when diagnosing patients with heel pain. It may also be due to a poor understanding of the pathophysiology of plantar heel spurs and/or plantar fasciitis by health professionals. The answer to the question is probably often "*Both*".

But when clinicians are asked which came first, this can be a little more difficult to answer. Let's start with definitions of the two conditions.

Heel spurs are defined as bony growths that extend from the skeleton into soft tissue (Benjamin et al 2006).

Plantar fasciitis has been traditionally defined as inflammation of the thick tissue (plantar
fascia) on the bottom of the foot. However Plantar 'fasciitis' is a misnomer since it is mostly a degenerative process, with little histological evidence of inflammation (Lemont et al 2003; Jarde et al 2003). Consequently, authors have termed it a fasciosis or fasciopathy since it encompasses both degenerative and inflammatory causes and is a general descriptor of pathology within the fascia. To discuss the semantics of the terminology is not the aim of this chapter and we shall leave this point here.

Heel Spur Pathophysiology

Osseous (bone) spurring of the plantar aspect of the calcaneus (heel) was first documented in 1900 by the German physician Plettner, who coined the term *Kalkaneussporn. Translation - calcaneal spur*. The pathophysiology of heel spurs is poorly understood. There are two popular reported hypotheses regarding the development of heel spurs.

Longitudinal traction hypothesis

It is hypothesised spurs may occur as a result of excessive repetitive traction by intrinsic muscles (small foot muscles), causing chronic microtrauma, which in turn, leads to periostitis (inflammation of the heel bone) and ossification (new bone growth). This is termed the *'longitudinal traction hypothesis' (Menz et al 2008). This hypothesis has been challenged due to* a number of study findings. In one study it was found that the bony trabeculae (direction of growth) of spurs are not aligned in the direction of soft tissue traction (Li & Muehleman 2007). Another study found that excised (surgical removed) spurs can reform after surgical release of the plantar fascia, however, symptoms of heel pain did not return (Tountas & Fornasier 1996).

Vertical compression hypothesis

An alternative hypothesis is the vertical compression hypothesis which suggests calcaneal spurs develop in response to repetitive compression rather than traction. Specifically, they suggest that calcaneal spurs are fibrocartilaginous outgrowths which form in response to calcaneal stress fractures, in an attempt to protect the calcaneus against microcracks (Kumai & Benjamin 2002). Moreover, the location of the calcaneal spurs on the deep surface of the plantar fascia suggests compression is the main stressor. In addition, Li and Muehleman (2007) have documented that the trabeculae within these calcaneal spurs are not oriented in the direction of soft-tissue traction but rather in a vertical orientation.

Body weight

There is a consensus among researchers that body weight may play a significant role in the development of heel spurs in that overweight individuals are more likely to develop heel spurs due to increased compression stress (Sedat-Ali 1998; Kaplan et al 2003; Bartold 2004; Menz et al 2008). Menz and colleagues (2008) found from 216 participants 45% classified as obese had heel spurs, compared to only 9% of those who were not obese.

Age

There is a fair level of evidence to suggest age plays a role in the development of heel spurs. A survey of 1,228 black Africans revealed that approximately 50% of patients who were more than 50 years of age had spurs. In the group of patients less than 30 years of age, the incidence dropped by 20%. A recent study including 1103 patients found a heel spur incidence rate of just 12.4% with that average age of the study group being 39 years of age.

Significance of heel spurs

The significance of a heel spur in patients with heel pain is a largely debated topic in podiatry. Heel spurs were originally considered to be an abnormality inextricably linked to heel pain. Even today, anecdotally, some General Practitioners, podiatrists, and physiotherapists believe that the plantar calcaneal spur causes plantar fasciitis pain, leading to referral for consideration of surgical removal of the spur (Johal & Milner 2012). On review of the literature, there is conflicting evidence regarding the significance of heel spurs in the role of plantar fasciitis. Some studies have reported a weak connection between heel spurs and plantar fasciitis whilst others have reported a strong link. It has been reported that the prevalence of heel spurs in the general population ranges from 8% to 18% (Shama et al 1983; Menz et al 2008). Shaman and colleagues (1983) reviewed 1000 radiographs and noted a 13.2% incidence of heel spurs but only 31% of these patients had symptoms of heel pain (Shama et al 1983). On the other hand, there are studies which found a high correlation between heel spurs and pain. Fakharian & Kalhor (2006) found in a sample of 625 that heel spurs developed in 33% of the general population and in nearly 80% of patients with painful heels. A recent study by Johal & Milner (2012) also found a significant association between heel spurs and plantar fasciitis (89%). It should be noted that this study was limited by a small population size (N=38).

In a large prospective study by Lee et al (2003) consisting of 435 patients with chronic proximal plantar fasciitis, 283 (65%) had an inferior calcaneal bone spur of variable size evident prior to treatment with high-energy extracorporeal shockwaves therapy. This included 308 patients who received ESWT and 127 placebo (not ESWT) patients. At both initial (3 months) and final (12 months) evaluations after receiving ESWT, no patient who received had significant disappearance or change in the radiographic appearance of the heel spur. Interestingly though, clinical outcome after ESWT was satisfactory in 168 patients (82%) with a radiographically demonstrable inferior heel spur and in 81 patients (79%) without such a heel spur. Therefore, the results showed no correlation between the presence or absence of the heel spur and the eventual treatment outcome. In essence, the presence or absence of a heel spur did not matter. Furthermore comparative surgical studies of plantar fascial release only vs heel spur resection with plantar fascial release reveal no major differences in outcome (Kinley et al 1993). Currently, to my knowledge, there is no evidence to prove a causal relationship between heel spurs and plantar fasciitis. furthermore, there is evidence against a causal link between plantar heel spurs and plantar fasciitis which comes from anatomical and MRI studies.

So which came first?

Although heel spurs have been described in association with plantar fasciitis, most publications conclude that they rarely cause this condition (Berkowitz 1991). Although a higher proportion of spurs is noted in plantar fasciitis, their presence is not causal. Plantar fasciitis may exist in the absence of a spur and asymptomatic spurs are common. It is believed that heel spurs develop secondary to plantar fasciitis as opposed to being a causative factor (Micke et al 2008).

Conclusion

What we do know is that age and body weight both play a significant role in the development of heel spurs. That is, they are particular more common in the older and obese populations. One theory to explain this pattern is that the development of heel spurs is a physiological (normal) process which happens very slowly over a lifetime and is thus not present until later years. It is the accumulation of physiological stress (normal weight bearing stress) being placed on the heels over the course of our lives which leads to the gradual development of heel spurs. It is evident that the prevalence of heel spurs in the younger population is very low by comparison regardless of whether they have plantar fasciitis or not. It is also known that obesity increases the compression stress on the heels which accelerates the *"Wear and tear"* of the heel bone leading to heel spurs in this population. Finally, heel spurs are overall undoubtedly more common in patients with plantar fasciitis than patients without plantar fasciitis. It is a logical notion that the causes of plantar fasciitis, a combination of traction stress and vertical stress will result overall in high levels of mechanical stress at the bottom of the heel. It is therefore of no surprise that heel spurs may develop secondary to these high-stress levels.

Tight Hamstrings Linked to Plantar Fasciitis

Over recent years there have been a number of studies demonstrating a link between tight hamstrings and plantar fasciitis. However, hamstring stretches are not a commonly prescribed exercise by clinicians for plantar fasciitis treatment. So we need to ask the question - **should the treatment plan also include hamstring stretches?**

Let's take a look...

Study 1

A study published in the journal, *Foot & Ankle Specialist* (2011) found that participants (86 of 210 feet) with hamstring tightness were 8.7 times as likely to experience plantar fasciitis as participants without hamstring tightness. Their study also found that patients with a Body Mass Index (BMI) greater than 35 were 2.4 times as likely as those with a BMI less than 35 to have plantar fasciitis. This also highlights the importance of weight loss as part of a patient's treatment plan if overweight and suffering from plantar fasciitis (Labovitz et al 2011).

study 2

A study, published in *Foot & Ankle International* looked at hamstring flexibility and forefoot loading stress. The results indicate that an increase in hamstring tightness may induce prolonged forefoot loading and through the windlass mechanism be a factor that increases repetitive injury to the plantar fascia (Harty et al 2005).

study 3

A more recent study also published in the journal *Foot & Ankle International* also found a significant relationship between tight hamstrings as well in tight calf muscles in plantar fasciitis sufferers in comparison to a control group of people who did not have plantar fasciitis and who had good hamstring a calf flexibility (Bolivar et al 2013).

Discussion

It is currently unclear as to how exactly the hamstrings play a role in plantar fasciitis. It has been suggested that an increase in hamstring tightness may induce prolonged forefoot loading and, through the windlass mechanism, may be a factor that increases repetitive plantar fascia injury.

Another possible cause may be the strong connection of the hamstrings to the calf muscles which then attach to the plantar fascia via the Achilles tendon. It is well known that an increase in tensile stress on the Achilles tendon transfers an increase in loading stress on the plantar fascia. Since the calf muscles are attached strongly to the hamstring via fascia (connective tissue) it is likely that any tightness in the hamstrings can transfer this tension down to the plantar fascia. This theory is supported by anatomical dissection studies completed by Thomas Myers published in his book 'Anatomy Trains' (2009) which demonstrate the strong connection running from the plantar fascia to knees and from the knees to the skull. This is known as the *superficial back line*.

Conclusion

It is well known that tight calf muscles are a causative factor in the development of plantar fasciitis. There have been a number of studies over the past 30 years to demonstrate this. Until recently, there has been a lack of studies looking at hamstring flexibility as another causative factor, however, these recent studies have now demonstrated a strong link. Therefore hamstring stretching exercises should play a crucial role in the treatment and prevention of plantar fasciitis. Below is a link to my exercise videos on stretching the superficial back line.

https://www.youtube.com/edit?o=U&video_id=qX7QwSTD-bE

https://www.youtube.com/edit?o=U&video_id=mJWNKhLT0Sk

https://www.youtube.com/edit?o=U&video_id=IJ2nWh3YS9k

Plantar Fascia Friendly Exercise

A commonly reported complaint from patients is that they cannot exercise due to their pain which contributes to weight gain. As being overweight has been identified as a risk factor for plantar fasciitis this causes a significant problem. There is a general consensus amongst health professionals that running is one of the worst exercises for aggravating plantar fasciitis. This is believed to be partly down to the high impact nature of running where the heel strikes the ground with a high magnitude of force along with the high levels of tensile stress placed on the plantar fascia to perform the biomechanical movement of running.

Alternative exercise

Patients that are wanting to exercise to keep up fitness levels or to lose weight whilst suffering from plantar fasciitis should try alternative exercises which do not aggravate plantar fasciitis or cause pain. Whilst this seems like common sense it is surprising how many patients are not aware of the potential delay in recovery they are causing when running and are unaware of safer and more suitable alternative exercises. Generally, lower impact exercise is usually less harmful such as:

Cycling - This is a low impact exercise. There is no weight directly placed on the heel minimising compressive stress over the plantar fascia. Cycling usually results in tightening of the calf muscles due to the repetitive concentric contraction of the calf muscles which can make plantar fasciitis worse, therefore it is important to stretch the calves thoroughly after cycling to minimise the negative effects of increased calf muscle tension.

Rowing - This is a low impact exercise and a good alternative exercise to running. Most gyms have indoor rowing machines. In terms of cardiovascular intensity, rowing is one of best exercises for increasing cardiovascular fitness and burning calories.

Cross trainer - this is a popular alternative to running and is a relatively low impact exercise. There is less impact placed directly on the heel during the elliptical motion on the cross trainer and therefore does not often cause aggravation of the plantar fascia. However, it is common for the back heel lift during forward motion via ankle plantarflexion which results in increased tensile loading of the plantar fascia and in some people this can aggravate their plantar fasciitis symptoms. If this is the case you should discontinue this exercise until a time when you can do it without pain.

Swimming - I have not heard of a case where a patient's plantar fasciitis symptoms have worsened due to swimming. As one is barefoot during swimming the foot is entirely unrestricted in its movements. The water provides a low level of resistance to fine muscle movements in the feet which may strengthen the foot muscles. This is why people often report cramping in the feet during and shortly after swimming, since the foot muscles are working exceptionally harder than they usually do and functioning in a different way, leading to fatigue and cramping. This is unlikely to have any negative effects on plantar fasciitis and there is some early stage evidence currently to suggest the importance of strong foot muscles in treating plantar fasciitis.

Prefabricated orthoses or custom made orthoses?

This is a question which is of particular interest to patients as it usually determines how much money they will end up spending on orthoses (insoles). To get to the point, both are very effective at treating plantar fasciitis. We know this based on the evidence base to prove their efficacy (see chapter four for more details). But what patients really want to know is whether custom-made orthoses are worth the extra expense?

There have been studies which have compared the efficacy of custom orthoses with that of prefabricated orthoses for treating plantar fasciitis. The research demonstrates that both are effective but there is not a significant difference between the two. Therefore from a cost effective point of view prefabricated orthoses are the better option. Having said that, there are a lot of variables such as the materials used to make both different types of orthoses.

There are literally hundreds of prefabricated orthoses on the market of which some are good and some are complete rubbish. It can be a minefield for patients when trying to select a prefabricated insole on the internet or in a shop which is a big problem with prefabricated orthoses. Prefabricated orthoses are not tailored to the patient's individual needs which are another potential limitation and thus can lead to suboptimal results.

Custom orthoses, however, provide an optimised level of functional support however this is influenced by the podiatrists prescription. There have been studies looking at prescription writing consistency between different podiatrists when treating the same patient which have found a poor inter-prescriber consistency meaning that each podiatrist writes the prescription differently. This is due to the difference in assessment techniques, levels of experience and difference of opinion amongst podiatrists. On one hand a podiatrist may prescribe a perfect orthotic device for a patient that really makes a difference above a prefabricated orthotic but on the other hand, another podiatrist may not achieve as great a success for another patient which may be down to the podiatrist's prescription choice.

My opinion - Personally I treat most patients with custom orthoses as a first line intervention as I feel I have seen great success rates with my patients in comparison to cases where I have prescribed prefabricated orthoses. Additionally, I also feel I am able to create a larger change in soft tissue stress which I believe to be of vital importance in treating plantar fasciitis successfully. Having said that I have found that some patients will also do well with prefabricated orthoses and do not require a more expensive custom made device but the success rate seems to be lower. In hindsight, I wish I had audited these patients!

Wearing a Night Splint

Night splints! Now, who actually enjoys wearing a night splint to bed? Absolutely no one.

People don't choose to wear night splints for comfort, let's face it, anything holding the foot in a certain position and restricting movement whilst we are trying to sleep isn't going to be the most enjoyable experience. So why do we recommend that patients wear night splints for plantar fasciitis?

To be to the point, they work. Tremendously well in fact. They significantly reduce pain first thing in the morning which allows the patient to start their day on the right foot (ahem pun intended). This also means the patient isn't re-injuring their heel every morning, allowing them to break the pain cycle and promote healing.

However, in my clinical experience, there appears to be a common theme amongst night splint wearers which is to over tighten the splint resulting in discomfort and noncompliance. This mistake is very easily made as it seems logical that the tighter the splint is the more stretch it is going to provide and after all isn't that exactly why the patient has been prescribed the night splint in the first place?

To explain why this is a problem I shall compare the stretch applied from a night splint with that compared to a static stretching exercise. When prescribing a stretching exercise clinicians usually ask the patient to hold the stretch for around 30 seconds and advise the patient that they should feel an intense stretch but not so much that it causes pain. This intense stretch is held for 30 seconds and rarely repeated more than 3 times, so that's 1:30 minutes worth a stretching. Now imagine holding that intense stretch for 8 hours. (if some of us are lucky to catch 8 hours sleep a night) As you can imagine an intense stretch held for this duration would begin to become very uncomfortable.

As the night splint is designed to be worn for around 8 hours continuously it is very unlikely to be tolerated if it is providing an intense stretch. A night splint is not designed for a high-intensity stretch. It is designed to provide a low grade, light stretch over a long duration. Even if it doesn't feel like it is providing much of a stretch at all it will still be serving a very important job which is preventing tightening of the calf muscles and plantar fascia during sleep. For nearly all of us, whilst we are sleeping the foot plantarflexes at the ankle (flexes downwards) which results in shortening of the calf muscles and plantar fascia. The problem with this is when the patient gets out of bed the next morning the ankle dorsiflexes in order to get the heel on the floor. This causes a very sudden change in the range of motion of the calf muscles in the opposite direction resulting in an increase in loading stress on the poor plantar fascia. Net result = PAIN!

Tip

For those of you that are struggling to wear your night splint, try loosening it. A loosely worn night splint is better than no splint at all. Here is a video on how the night splint works.

More on Trigger Point Therapy

Trigger point therapy has become increasingly popular over recent years in the UK and is currently the hot topic for relieving a wide range of musculoskeletal pain including plantar fasciitis. I have therefore felt the need to discuss trigger point therapy in more detail. This article is by no means a thorough explanation of the history and philosophy of trigger point therapy but should serve to give a brief overview and more importantly explain how it can help treat plantar fasciitis.

Trigger point therapy has been around since 1942 where it was first coined by Dr. J Travell following her work on myofascial pain syndrome. Myofascial pain syndrome is described as hyperirritable areas associated within a taut band of a skeletal muscle that is painful on compression, contraction, or stretching of the muscles, and elicit a referred pain distant to the trigger point (Simons et al 1999).

How Do I get Trigger Points?

It is believed that they are established by the trauma that occurs during injury from accidents, sports, occupations, and disease. They can also be caused by long-term or repetitive strain on muscles from poor ergonomics, posture and repetitive movements. It is also believed that physical or emotional stress frequently aggravate trigger points. Finally, it is reported that myofascial pain accounts for as much as 85% of the pain people suffer from and that acute and chronic myofascial pain due to trigger points is a very common condition.

Trigger point controversy

The Western medical community at large has not embraced trigger point therapy. Although trigger points do appear to be an observable phenomenon with defined properties, there is a lack of a consistent methodology for diagnosing trigger points. A systematic review conducted by Lucas and colleagues (2009) scrutinised 9 papers on the clinical diagnosis of trigger points. Their conclusion below highlights key areas of concern which serve as large barriers for trigger point therapy to gain respect within Western medicine.

'No study to date has reported the reliability of trigger point diagnosis according to the currently proposed criteria. On the basis of the limited number of studies available, and significant problems with their design, reporting, statistical integrity, and clinical applicability, physical examination cannot currently be recommended as a reliable test for the diagnosis of trigger points. The reliability of trigger point diagnosis needs to be further investigated with studies of high quality that use current diagnostic

criteria in clinically relevant patients.'

This does not mean that trigger point therapy is pseudoscience but instead points out that clinical examination alone is not a reliable method for diagnosing trigger points. However, an interesting study by Chen et al (2007) has found that the stiffness of trigger point taut bands was 50% greater than that of the surrounding muscle tissues when objectively investigated using magnetic resonance elastography (MRE). This provides some evidence into the legitimacy of myofascial trigger points within the body. It should be pointed out that the findings of this study are limited as they only used two participants.

How does trigger point therapy work?

It is believed that trigger point therapy allows your body to undergo soft tissue release, allowing for increased blood flow, a reduction in muscle spasm, and the break-up of scar tissue. It is believed to help remove any build-up of toxic metabolic waste.

Trigger point therapy for plantar fasciitis

Although there is considerable anecdotal evidence, currently there is a paucity of clinical research evidence to support the use of trigger point therapy, however, one particular study looked at trigger point therapy in the management of plantar fasciitis.

A randomized clinical control trial (gold standard research) compared two groups of patients - trigger point therapy and stretching vs stretching alone. Patients receiving a combination of self-stretching and Trigger point therapy intervention showed a greater improvement in Pressure pain thresholds, as compared to those who received only the self-stretching protocol.

empowering self-care

Although patients are unable to duplicate therapy outside of clinics due to its specific nature and expertise provided by seeing a health professional, a self-applied trigger point is a conduit between your clinic and your home which is now made easily achievable thanks to Trigger Point Performance™ who have designed a self-treatment kit. This treatment kit allows you to self-treat your plantar fasciitis from home and will reduce the amount of clinical time you need to spend with a health professional to perform trigger point therapy for you. It is equally important for patients to be actively involved in their rehabilitation. Patients need to take responsibility for managing their own care. From time to time, of course, you may find you need help from medical professionals. But even so, the more you know, the better care you're going to receive. This is naturally going to require some time and effort on your part, but the payoff will be faster with far better results.

Conclusion

Regardless of whether myofascial pain syndrome truly exists or whether there are specific trigger points within the body or not. Trigger point therapy can be used effectively is an additional method to loosen tight calf muscles. They are an excellent adjunct along with a traditional stretching programme to make further gains in flexibility and a speedier recovery from plantar fasciitis. As this is a simple and safe treatment it is highly recommended!

Leg Length Discrepancy and Plantar Fasciitis

The development of plantar fasciitis is believed to be mechanical. The plantar fascia is a strong and tough connective tissue that is designed to withstand high levels of mechanical stress. There are many reasons why the plantar fascia might be subject to increased levels of stress including muscular tightness of the calves and hamstrings, excess foot pronation etc. Here I would like to give a brief mention to leg length discrepancy as a causative factor for increased mechanical stress on the plantar fascia which may lead to plantar fasciitis.

Leg length discrepancy greater than 2cm is reported to affect 1 in 1000 people (Mahmood et al 2010). It is widely accepted that compensations by the body occur to lengthen the short leg and shorten the long leg in an attempt to provide a 'balance', however the nature of these compensations varies.

Leg length discrepancy can for into two types:

1 - structural, this means a shortening of the skeleton

2 - functional, this means the skeleton is equal in length to left and right, however, a discrepancy occurs due to altered mechanics of the lower legs

For an efficient move to occur, proper symmetry and alignment of the body are necessary. If asymmetry exists, in particular by leg length discrepancy, then gait and posture are disrupted and symptoms can occur (Mahmood et al 2010).

There is a lack of clinical research looking at leg length discrepancy is an isolated cause of heel pain, however, Mahmood and colleagues (2010) investigated 26 patients diagnosed with plantar fasciitis. They used a combination of methods to measure leg lengths in order to improve the accuracy of measurement. They found that 87.5% of patients with left heel pain measured the left leg being the longer side and that 93.3% of patients with right heel pain measured the right leg being the longer side. These findings indicate a strong correlation between a longer leg and plantar fasciitis pain.

On the other hand, it should be made clear that the quality of this study is rather poor due to a small sample size of the patient and the methods used for measuring leg length difference are have been shown to be unreliable. Furthermore, this study demonstrates a strong correlation but it does not demonstrate causation.

Recommendations

It is recommended that clinicians should assess for a leg length discrepancy routinely when performing a physical examination of patients with heel pain and consider the clinical relevance of this on an individual basis. Future research into leg length discrepancy as a causative factor needs to be conducted so that patients and clinicians can be better guided on the relevance of a leg length discrepancy.

Plantar Fasciitis Treatment Pathway

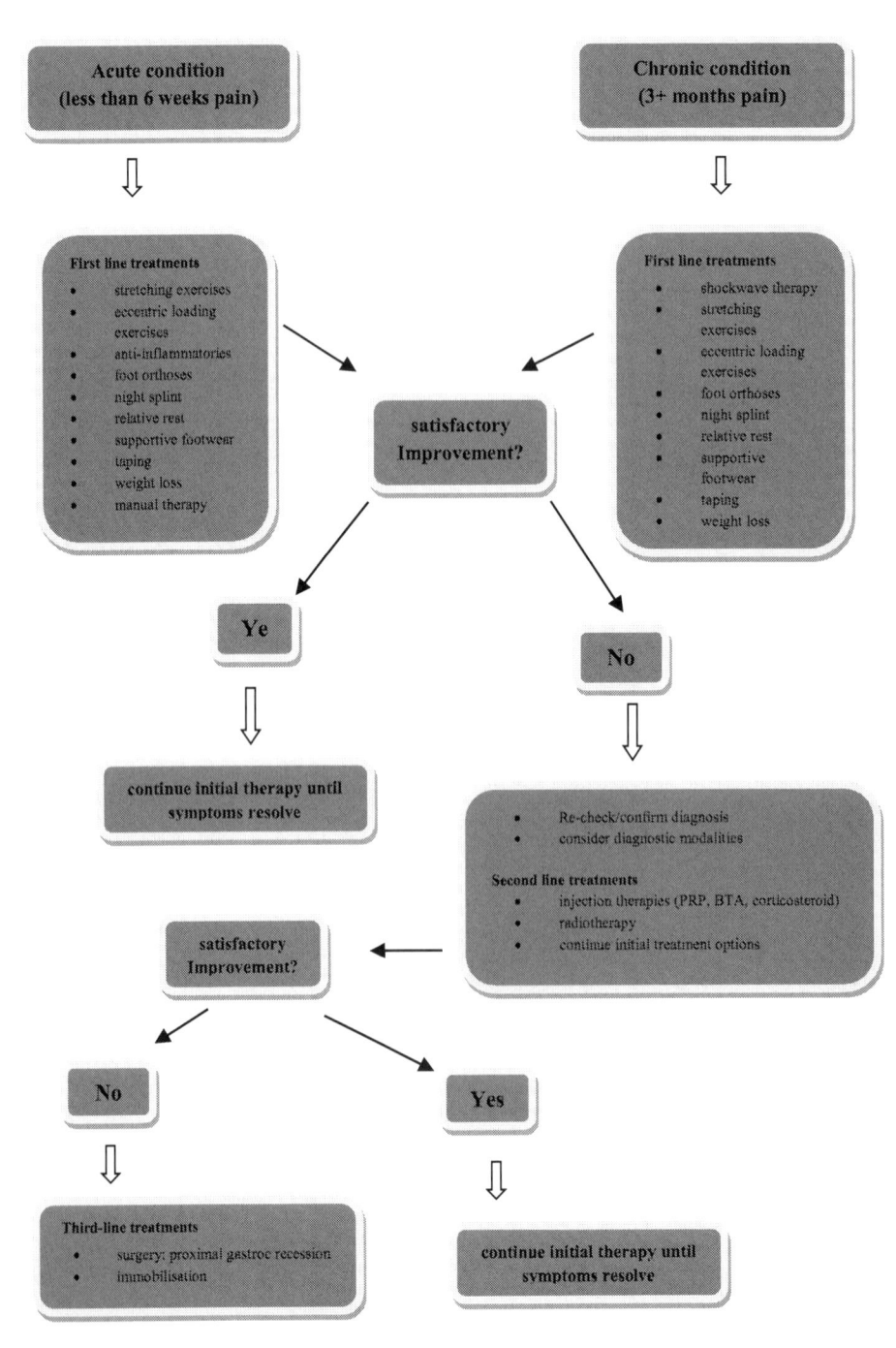

Acute condition (less than 6 weeks pain)

First line treatments
- stretching exercises
- eccentric loading exercises
- anti-inflammatories
- foot orthoses
- night splint
- relative rest
- supportive footwear
- taping
- weight loss
- manual therapy

Chronic condition (3+ months pain)

First line treatments
- shockwave therapy
- stretching exercises
- eccentric loading exercises
- foot orthoses
- night splint
- relative rest
- supportive footwear
- taping
- weight loss

satisfactory Improvement?

Yes → continue initial therapy until symptoms resolve

No →
- Re-check/confirm diagnosis
- consider diagnostic modalities

Second line treatments
- injection therapies (PRP, BTA, corticosteroid)
- radiotherapy
- continue initial treatment options

satisfactory Improvement?

No → Third-line treatments
- surgery: proximal gastroc recession
- immobilisation

Yes → continue initial therapy until symptoms resolve

Chapter Ten

Final Thoughts

Podiatrists aren't the only health professionals that diagnose and treat plantar fasciitis. This common condition is also seen by a wide network of professionals including GP's, physiotherapists, sports therapists, chiropractors, osteopaths, sports medicine physicians, rheumatologists, and orthopaedic surgeons. Currently, there is a lack of consensus on how to manage this common condition amongst different health professionals. This is influenced by the underpinning philosophy of healthcare within each profession. For instance, an osteopath may take a more 'hands-on' manual therapy approach such as soft tissue mobilisation techniques to release tight muscles associated with the condition. A chiropractor may perform joint manipulations in an attempt to restore normal foot function. A podiatrist may prescribe foot orthoses in an attempt to biomechanically reduce soft tissue stress on the plantar fascia. A physiotherapist may try acupuncture and a prescribed exercise programme. An orthopaedic surgeon may provide a corticosteroid injection or surgical release of the plantar fascia. There is also a large overlap in treatment interventions amongst different health professionals as most will also provide stretching exercises along with other treatments such as massage, laser therapy etc. Each of these different professions reports having overall success in managing plantar fasciitis, often applying methods which work best for them anecdotally based on their own individual experience. In order to improve the consistency of success, it is of paramount importance that professionals provide **evidence-informed treatment**. That is treatments which are supported or influenced by high-quality research evidence. This is a key driver for the future of successful healthcare. In modern healthcare it is no longer acceptable for professionals to remain ignorant to evidence-based medicine, applying treatments which have poor evidence to support their use. Professionals need not abandon what they are taught traditionally during their training but to think critically and to question the underpinning philosophy they are taught on how we manage plantar fasciitis, asking *"is this evidence-informed treatment?"*

An example of applying critical thinking can be found amongst the podiatry profession. It was originally taught as part of a podiatrists training that there is an ideal structure of the foot that tends to allow the most normal function during weight bearing activities.

This thinking was based on the theory of Merton Root (1971), commonly known as the subtalar joint neutral theory. In the subtalar neutral theory, any foot that stood pronated or supinated from the neutral position was considered to be *"Abnormally pronated or supinated."*

Therefore the aim of treatment utilising this theory was to restore subtalar neutral alignment via foot orthoses (insoles). Whilst this theory produced good treatment results for many patients, podiatrists have moved away from this theory of mechanical foot therapy due to some inherent problems and inconsistencies highlighted by more modern biomechanical research such as that conducted by McPoil & Cornwall (1994). As a result of the highlighted flaws with the Root theory, a new model was proposed in 1995 by McPoil and Hunt - *the tissue stress model* (see Chapter 8). This new model has changed to way podiatrists prescribe foot orthoses which have led to improvements in patient care. This model is still widely accepted today amongst an array of health professionals and scientists. This is just one example of a profession applying critical thinking to traditional philosophy which has led to an improvement in patient care and I do not doubt that there have been other developments within other professions over the past 40 years. The take home message is that evidence-based medicine is a continuous evolutionary process and every health professional in each profession needs to keep up to date with the latest research, focus their treatment plan on evidence-based medicine and discontinue treatments which have been proven to have a poor evidence base.

Bibliography

Acevedo J, Besin J. (1998) Complications of plantar fascia rupture associated with corticosteroid injections. *Foot Ankle Int.* Volume 19:91–97

Aksahin E et al (2012). The comparison of the effect of corticosteroids and platelet-rich plasma (PRP) for treatment of plantar fasciitis. Arch Orthop Trauma Surg. Volume 132, pp 781-785

Alshami A M, Souvlis T., Coppieters MW., A review of plantar heel pain of neural origin: Differential diagnosis and management. Manual Therapy Volume 13, Issue 2, April 2008, Pages 103–111

Androsoni R., Apostolico Netto A., Rocha Macedo R., Pozzi Fasolin R., Boni G., Fileto R., Moreira G. (2013). Treatment of chronic plantar fasciitis with extra corporeal shock wave therapy: ultrasonographic morphological aspect and functional evaluation. Rev Bras Ortop.Volume 48(6): 538-544

American Physical Therapy Association. (2014). Heel Pain - Plantar Fasciitis: Revision 2014 Journal of Orthopaedic & Sports Physical Therapy. Volume 44. Number 11

Arenson, DJ (1980) The inferior calcaneal nerve: an anatomical study Journal of the American Podiatry Association, 70 (11), pp.

552–560

Arnett FC, Edworthy SM, Bloch DA, et al. (1998) The American Rheumatism Association 1987 revised criteria for the classification of rheumatoid arthritis. *Arthritis Rheum.* Volume 31:315–324

Attard J & Singh D. (2012). A comparison of two night ankle-foot orthoses used in the treatment of inferior heel pain: a preliminary investigation. Foot & Ankle Surgery. Volume 18 (2): 108-10

Babcock M., Foster L., Pasquina P., Jabbari B. (2005). Treatment of pain attributed by plantar fasciitis with botulinum toxin A: a short term randomised, placebo-controlled, double blinded study. AM J Phys Med Rehabil. Vol 84 (9):649-654

Badakhshi H and Buadch. (2014). Low dose radiotherapy for plantar fasciitis. Treatment outcome of 171 patients. The Foot. Volume 24, Issue 4, Pages 172-175

Banadda BM et al (1992) Calcaneal spurs in a Black African population. Foot Ankle Int, 13. pp. 352–354

Berkowitz JF, Kier R, Rudicel S. (1991) Plantar fasciitis: MR imaging. *Radiology.* Volume 179:665–667

Bartold SJ. (2004). The plantar fascia as a source of pain—biomechanics, presentation and treatment. Journal of Bodywork and Movement Therapies. Volume 8:214–26.

Baker KG., Robertson VJ., Duck FA. (2001). A review of therapeutic ultrasound: biophysical effects. Phys Ther. 81(7):1351-8

Barrett S.L., Day S.V., Pignetti T.T., Robinson L.B. (1995). Endoscopic plantar fasciotomy: A multi-surgeon prospective analysis of 652 cases. J Foot Ankle Surg. Volume 34:400–406

Barry LD., Barry AN., Chen Y. (2002). A retrospective study of standing gastrocnemius-soleus stretching versus night splinting in the treatment of plantar fasciitis. Journal of Foot & Ankle Surgery. Volume 41 (4): 221-7

Baxter D.E., Pfeffer GB. (1992). Treatment of chronic heel pain by surgical release of the first branch of the lateral plantar nerve. Clinical Orthopaedics and Related Research (279) (1992), pp. 229–236

Bedi DG and Davidson DM. (2001). Plantar Fibromatosis: Most Common Sonographic Appearance and Variations. Journal of Clinical Ultrasound. Volume 29. 449-501.

Benjamin M, Toumi H, Ralphs J, Bydder G, Best T, Milz S. (2006). Where tendons and ligaments meet bone: attachment sites ('entheses') in relation to exercise and/or mechanical load. Journal of Anatomy. Volume 208:471–90.

Bluestone R. (1982). Collagen diseases affecting the foot. *Foot Ankle.* Volume 2:311–317

Bolivar YA., Munuera PV., Padillo JP. (2013). Relationship Between Tightness of the Posterior Muscles of the Lower Limb and Plantar Fasciitis. Foot Ankle Int, January 2013; vol. 34, 1: pp. 42-48.

Bolgla LA and Malone T. (2004). Plantar Fasciitis and the Windlass Mechanism: A Biomechanical Link to Clinic Practice. Journal of Athletic Training. Volume 39 (1): 77-82

Buchbinder R et al. (2002). Ultrasound-guided extracorporeal shock wave therapy for plantar fasciitis. JAMA. Volume 288: 136472.
Campbell JW and Inman VT. (1974). Treatment of plantar fasciitis and calcaneal spurs with the UC-BL shoe insert. Clinical

Orthopaedics and Related Research. (103): 57-62

Carlson RE., Fleming LL., Hutton WC. (2000). The Biomechanical Relationship Between The Tendoachilles, Plantar Fascia and Metatarsophalangeal Joint Dorsiflexion Angle. Foot & Ankle International. Vol 21, 1: pp 18-25

Chen Q, Bensamoun S, Basford JR, Thompson JM, A KN. (2007) Identification and quantification of myofascial taut bands with magnetic resonance elastography. Arch Phys Med Rehabil. Volume 88:1658-166

Chuckpaiwong B, Berkson EM, Theodore GH. (2009) Extracorporeal shock wave for chronic proximal plantar fasciitis: 225 patients with results and outcome predictors. J Foot Ankle Surg. Volume 48:148–55

Christman RA. (2003) Foot and ankle radiology. St. Louis: Churchill Livingston.

Crane JD., Ogborn DI., Cupido C., Melov S., Hubbard A., Bourgeois JM., Tarnopolsky MA. (2012). Massage therapy attenuates inflammatory signaling after exercise-induced muscle damage. Sci Trans Med. Volume 1;4 (119).

Davis PF, Sevrerind E, Baxter DE. (1994) Painful heel syndrome: results of non-operative treatment. Foot Ankle, 17: 527-532

Dellon AL. (1996) Computer-assisted sensibility evaluation and surgical treatment of the tarsal tunnel syndrome. *Adv Podiatr Med Surg*;2:17–40

Diaz-Llopis IV., Rodriquez-Ruiz CM., Mulet-Perry S., Mondejar-Gomez FJ., Climent-Barbera JM., Cholbi-Llobel F. (2012). Randomised controlled study of the efficacy of the injection of botulinum toxin type A versus corticosteroids in chronic plantar fasciitis: results at one and six months. Clinical Rehabilitation. Vol 26 (7): 594-606.

Díaz-Llopis IV, Gómez-Gallego D, Mondéjar-Gómez FJ, López-García A, Climent-Barberá JM, Rodríguez-Ruiz CM. **(2013). Botulinum toxin type A in chronic plantar fasciitis: clinical effects one year after injection.** Clin Rehabil. **Vol 27(8):681-5**

DiGiovanni BF., Nawoczenski DA., Lintal ME., Moore EA. Murray JC., Wilding GE., Baumhauer JF. (2003). Tissue-specific plantar fascia-stretching exercise enhances outcomes in patients chronic heel pain. A prospective, randomized study. Journal of Bone & Joint Surgery American Edition. Volume 85 -A (7): 1270-7

Elizondo-Rodriguez J., Araujo-Lopez Y., Moreno-Gonzalez JA., Cardenas-Estrada E., Mendoza-Lemus O., Acosta-Olivo C. (2013). A comparison botulinum toxin A and intralesional steroids for the treatment of plantar fasciitis: A randomised, double blinded study. Foot & Ankle International. Vol 34 (1) 8-14.

Fakharian M, Kalhor M. (2006). A Comparative Study of Heel Spur Incidence in Patients with Painful Heels and General Population Over Forty Years. RJMS. Volume 12 (49) :137-144

Falsetti P, Frediani B, Acciai C, et al (2004) Heel fat pad involvement in rheumatoid arthritis and in spondyloarthropathies: an ultrasonographic study. *Scand J Rheumatol.* Volume 33:327–331

Faria A, Gabriel R, Abrantes J, Brás R, Moreira H. (2009). Tricepssurae musculotendinous stiffness: relative differences between obese and non-obese postmenopausal women. Clin Biomech. Volume. 24(10):866–871

Fishco WD, Stiles RG**.** Atypical heel pain. (1999) Hyperparathyroidism induced stress fracture of the calcaneus.

J Am Podiatr Med Assoc. Volume 89:413–418

Flanigan RM., Nawoczenski DA., Chen L., Wu H., DiGiovanni BF. (2007). The Influence of Foot Position and Stretching of the Plantar Fascia. Foot & Ankle International. Vol 28,7: pp 815-822

Franceschi F., Papalia R., Franceschetti E., Paciott M., Maffuli N., Denaro V. (2014). Platelet-rich plasma injections for chronic plantar fasciopathy: a systematic review British Medica Bulletin

<u>Franson J and Baravarian B (2006). Tarsal Tunnel Syndrome: A Compression Neuropathy Involving Four Distinct Tunnels. Clinics in Podiatric Medicine and Surgery. Volume 23, Issue 3, Pages 597-609</u>

Frey C and Zamora J. (2007). The effect of obesity on orthopaedic foot and ankle pathology. Foot & Ankle International. Volume 28 (9): 996-9

Gollwitzer H, Diehl P, von Korff A, et al. (2007). Extracorporeal shock wave therapy for chronic painful heel syndrome: a prospective, double-blind, randomized trial assessing the efficacy of a new electromagnetic shock wave device. J Foot Ankle Surg. Volume 46:348–57

Gray H et al (2005). Anatomy: the anatomical basis of clinical practice (39th ed)Elsevier Churchill Livingstone, Edinburgh (2005)

Harty J., Soffe K., O'Toole G., Stephens MM. (2005). Foot Ankle Int. Volume 26(12):p 1089-1092

Hendrix et al (1998) Entrapment neuropathy: the etiology of intractable chronic heel pain syndrome The Journal of Foot and Ankle Surgery, 37 (4), pp. 273–279
Huang YC., Wei SH., Wang HK., Lieu FK. (2010).

Ultrasonographic guided botulinum toxin type A treatment for plantar fasciitis: an outcome-based investigation for treating pain and gait changes. Journal of Rehabilitation Medicine. Vol 42 (2): 136-40

Harty J., Soffe K., O'Toole G., Stephens MM. (2005). Foot Ankle Int, December 2005; vol. 26, 12: pp. 1089-1092

Healey K., Chen K. (2010). Plantar Fasciitis: Current Diagnostic Modalities and Treatments. Clinics in Podiatric Medicine and Surgery. Volume 27, Issue 3, p 369-380

Heyd R, Tselis N, Ackermann H, et al. (2007). Radiation therapy for painful heel spurs. Strahlentherapie und Onkologie. 183: 3-9

Hicks JH. (1954) The mechanics of the foot. II. The plantar aponeurosis and the arch.

J Anat. 1954 Jan;88(1):25-30.

Ieong E et al (2013). Ultrasound scanning for recalcitrant plantar fasciopathy. Basis of a new classification. Skeletal Radiology. Volume 42(3):393-8

Jarde O, Diebold P, Havet E, Boulu G, Vernois J. (2003) Degenerative lesions of the plantar fascia: surgical treatment by fasciectomy and excision of the heel spur. A report on 38 cases. Acta Orthop Belg 2003: 69: 267–274.

Johal KS and Milner SA. (2012). Plantar Fasciitis and the calcaneal spur: Fact or fiction? Foot and Ankle Surgery. 18.p 31-41

Kaplan MS, Huguet N, Newsom JT, McFarland BH, Lindsay J (2003): Prevalence and correlates of overweight and obesity among older adults: findings from the Canadian National Population Health Survey. *J Gerontol A Biol Sci Med Sci.* Volume

58(11): M1018-1030.

Kinley S, Frascone S, Calderone D et al. (1993). Endoscopic plantar fasciotomy versus traditional heel spur surgery: a prospective study: Journal of Foot and Ankle Surgery. Volume 32 p 305-311

Kibler WB, Goldberg C, Chandler TJ. (1991). Functional biomechanical deficits in running athletes with plantar fasciitis. Am J Sports Med. Volume 19:66–71

Kirby KA (2009). Foot and Lower Extremity Biomechanics, Vol IV: Precision Intricast Newsletters, 2009-2013.

Klippel JH, Stone JH, Crofford LJ, et al. **Primer on the rheumatic diseases.** 13th edition. New York: Arthritis Foundation; 2008;

Kogler GF, Veer FB, Solomonidis SE, Paul JP (1999). The influence of medial and lateral placement of orthotic wedges on loading of the plantar aponeurosis. J Bone Joint Surg Am. Volume 81:1403–1413.

Kopell HP and Thompson WA. (1960). Peripheral entrapment neuropathies of the lower extremity The New England Journal of Medicine, 14 (262) pp. 56–60

Kumai T, Benjamin M (2002). Heel spur formation and the subcalcaneal enthesis of the plantar fascia. *J Rheumatol.* Volume 29:1957-1964

Labovitz JM., Jenny Y., Kim C. (2011). Foot Ankle Specialist. Vol. 4, 3: pp. 141-144

Landorf KB, Keenan AM, Herbert RD. (2006) The effectiveness of foot orthoses to treat plantar fasciitis: a randomized trial. *Arch Intern Med* 2006;166:1305–1310.

Langberg H, Ellingsgaard H, Madsen T, Jansson J, Magnusson SP, Aagaard P, Kjaer M. (2007) Eccentric rehabilitation exercise increases peritendinous type I collagen synthesis in humans with Achilles tendinosis. Scand J Med Sci Sports 2007: 17: 61–66

Leach R, Jones R, Silva T. (1978) Rupture of the plantar fascia in athletes. *J Bone Joint Surg Am*;60:537–539

Lemont H, Ammirati KM, Usen N. (2003) Plantar fasciitis. A degenerative process (fasciosis) without inflammation. J Am Podiatr Med Assoc. Volume 93(3):234-237.

Langberg H, Ellingsgaard H, Madsen T, Jansson J, Magnusson SP, Aagaard P, Kjaer M. (2007) Eccentric rehabilitation exercise increases peritendinous type I collagen synthesis in humans with Achilles tendinosis. Scand J Med Sci Sports. Volume 17: 61–66

Li J., Muehleman C. (2007).Anatomic relationship of heel spur to surrounding soft tissues: greater variability than previously reported. *Clin Anat*. Volume 20:950-955.

Lichniak JE. (1990) The heel in systemic disease. *Clin Podiatr Med Surg*. 7:225–241

Lee GP., Ogden JA., Cross GL. (2003). Effect of extracorporeal shock waves on calcaneal bone spurs. Foot & Ankle International. volume 24 (12):9270-30

Louisia S and Masquelet AC. (1999) The medial and inferior calcaneal nerves: an anatomic study Surgical and Radiologic Anatomy, 21 (3), pp. 169–173

Lucas N., Macaskill P., Irwig L., Moran R., Bogduk K. (2009). Reliability of physical examination for diagnosis of myofascial trigger points: a systematic review of the literature. The Clinical Journal of Pain. Volume 25 (1): 80-9.
Lui E. Systemic Causes of Heel Pain. (2010). Clinics in Podiatric

Medicine and Surgery Volume 27, Issue 3, Pages 431-441

Lynch DM., Goforth WP., Martin JE., Odom RD., Preece CK., Kotter MW. (1998). Conservative treatment of plantar fasciitis. A prospective study: J Am Podiatr Med Assoc. 88(8):375-80.

Mahmood S, Huffman LK, Harris JG. (2010). Limb-Length Discrepancy as a Causes of Plantar Fasciitis. JAPMA. Volume 100. No 6.

Malay DS, Pressman MM, Assili A, et al. (2006). Extracorporeal shockwave therapy versus placebo for the treatment of chronic proximal plantar fasciitis: results of a randomized, placebo-controlled, double-blinded, multicenter intervention trial. J Foot Ankle Surg. Volume 45:196–210

Marks W, Jackiewicz A, Witkowski Z, et al. (2008). Extracorporeal shock-wave therapy (ESWT) with a new-generation pneumatic device in the treatment of heel pain. A double blind randomised controlled trial. Acta Orthop Belg. Volume 74:98–10

Menz HB., Zammit GV., Landorf K., Munteanu SE. (2008). Plantar calcaneal spurs in older people: longitudinal traction or vertical compression Journal of Foot and Ankle Research, 1, p. 7

Micke O, Ernst-Stecken A, Mücke R, et al. Calcaneodynia (2008). plantar and dorsal heel spur/heel spur syndrome. In: Seegenschmiedt MH, Makoski HB, Trott KR, et al., editors. Radiotherapy for Nonmalignant Disorders. Berlin: Springer. p. 295-315.

Monto RR. (2014). Platelet-rich plasma efficacy versus corticosteroid injection treatment for chronic severe plantar fasciitis. Foot & Ankle International. Volume 35(4):313-8

Murphy, PC and Baxter DE. (1985) Nerve entrapment of the foot and ankle in runners. Clinics in Sports Medicine, 4 (4), pp. 753–763

Myers TW.(2009). Anatomy Trains. Myofascial Meridians for Manual and Movement Therapists. Second edition. Churchill Livingstone. Elsevier.

McMillan AM, Landorf KB, Gilheany MF, et al. (2012). Ultrasound guided corticosteroid injection for plantar fasciitis: randomised controlled trial. BMJ. 344:e3260

McPoil TG., Cornwall MW. (1994). the relationship between subtalar joint neutral position and rearfoot motion during walking. Foot & Ankle International. Volume 15. p 141-145.

Niewald M., Seegenschmiedt MH, Micke O., Graeber S., Muecke R., Schaefer V., Scheid C., Fleckenstein J., Licht N. Ruebe C. (2012). Randomized, Multicenter Trial on the Effect of Radiation Therapy on Plantar Fasciitis (Painful Heel Spur) Comparing a Standard Dose With a Very Low Dose: Mature Results After 12 Months' Follow-Up. Radiation Oncology International Journal of biology physics No. pp. 1e8, 2012

O'Brien D, Martin WJ (1985) A retrospective analysis of heel pain. J Am Podiatr Med Assoc 75: 416-418.

Ozkaya & Nihat (1999). Stress and Strain. IN: Leger DL. Fundamentals of Biomechanics: Equilibrium, Motion, and Deformation. Springer Publishing

Oztuna V et al (2002). Nerve entrapment in painful heel syndrome. Foot and Ankle International, 23 (3) pp. 208–211

Patel A., DiGiovanni B. (2011). Association between plantar fasciitis and isolated contracture of the gastrocnemius. Foot & Ankle International. Volume 32 (1): 5-8

Peterlein CD., Funk JF., Holscher A., Schuh A., Placzek R. (2012). Is botulinum toxin effective for the treatment of plantar fasciitis?

Clinical Journal of Pain. Vol 28 (6): 527-533

Porter D, Barrill E., Oneacre K., and May BD. (2002). The Effects of Duration and Frequency of Achilles Tendon Stretching on Dorsiflexion and Outcome in Painful Heel Syndrome: A Randomized, Blinded, Control Study. Foot and ankle International. Volume 23: 619.
Raikin SM and Schon LC. (2000) Nerve entrapment in the foot and ankle of an athlete Sports Medicine and Arthroscopy Review, 8 (4) pp. 387–394
Rajput B, Abboud RJ. Common ignorance, major problem: the role of footwear in plantar fasciitis. Foot. 2004;14:214–218

Reade BM, Longo DC, Keller MC. (2001) **Tarsal tunnel syndrome.** *Clin Podiatr Med Surg;*18(3):395–408

Renan-Ordine R et al (2011). The effectiveness of myofascial trigger point manual therapy combined with a self-stretching protocol for the management of plantar heel pain: randomized controlled trial. J Orthop Sports Phys Ther. Volume 41(2):43-50

Robert E., Carlson MD and Lamar L. (2000). The Biomechanical Relantionship Between the Tendoachilles, Plantar Fascia and Metatarsophalangeal Joint Dorsiflexion Angle. Foot & Ankle International. Volume 21. No 2

Rome K, Howe T, Haslock I. (2001) Risk factors associated with the development of plantar heel pain in athletes. The Foot. Volume 11(3):119-125.

Root ML., Orien WP., Weed JH., Hughes RJ. (1971). Biomechanical Examination of the Foot, Volume 1. Clinical Biomechanics Corporation, Los Angeles.

Resnick D, Feingold MS, Curd J, et al. Calcaneal abnormalities in articular disorders, rheumatoid arthritis, ankylosing spondylitis, psoriatic arthritis and Reiter's syndrome. *Radiology.*

1977;125:355–366

Rathleff MS., Molgaard CM., Fredberg U., Kaalund S., Anderson KB., Jensen TT., Aaskov S., Olesen JL. (2014). High-load strength training improved outcome in patients with plantar fasciitis: A randomized controlled trial with 12-month follow up. Scandinavian Journal of Medicine & Science in Sports. doi: 10.1111/sms.12313

Rondhuis JJ., A. Huson A. (1986) The first branch of the lateral plantar nerve and heel pain Acta Morphologica Neerlando-Scandinavica, 24 (4) pp. 269–279

Rothschild BM, Sebes JI. (1981). Calcaneal abnormalities and erosive bone disease associated with sickle cell anemia. *Am J Med*.71:427–430

Roos E., Engstrom M., Soderberg B. (2006). Foot orthoses for the treatment of plantar fasciitis. Foot & Ankle International. vol. 27 no. 8 606-611

Roxas M. (2005). Plantar fasciitis: diagnosis and therapeutic considerations. Altern Med Rev. 10(2):83-93

Sadat-Ali M (1998). Plantar fasciitis/calcaneal spur among security forces personnel.

Mil Med. Volume 163:56-57

Saxelby J et al (1997). An Assessment of the effectiveness of low dye stapping on the foot in the management of Plantar Fasciitis. The Foot: International Journal of Clinical Foot Science, 7, pp. 205-209

Saxena A, Fullem B. (2004). Plantar fascia ruptures in athletes. *Am J Sports Med.* Volume 32:662–665

Schon et al (1993). Heel pain syndrome: electrodiagnostic support for nerve entrapment Foot and Ankle, 14 (3), pp. 129–135

Sellman JR. (1994). Plantar fascia rupture associated with corticosteroid injection. Foot & Ankle International. Volume 15(7):376-81

Shama SS., Kominsky SJ., Lamont H., (1983) Prevalence of non-painful heel spur and its relation to postural foot position. Journal of the American Podiatry Association. Volume 73: 122-123

Shetty VD et al (2014). A study to compare the efficacy of corticosteroid therapy with platelet-rich plasma therapy in recalcitrant plantar fasciitis: a preliminary report. Foot & Ankle Surgery. Volume 20(1), pp 10-13

Simons DG, Travell JG, Simons LS. (1999) Travell & Simons' myofascial pain and dysfunction: the trigger point manual. 2nd ed. Williams & Wilkins; Baltimore:
Speed C. (2012*). A systematic review of shockwave therapies in soft tissue conditions: focusing on the evidence. BJSM.* Volume 48, Issue 21

Stecco C, Corradin M, Macchi V, Morra A, Porzionato A, Biz C, De Caro R. (2013). Plantar fascia anatomy and its relationship with Achilles tendon and paratenon. Journal of Anatomy 223: 665–676

Surenkok S., Dirican B., Beyzadeoglu M., Oysul K. (2006). Heel spur radiotherapy and radiation carcinogenesis risk estimation. Radiation Medicine. Volume 24, Issue 8: pp 573-576

Tountas AA, Fornasier VL (1996) Operative treatment of subcalcaneal pain. *Clin Orthop Relat Res.* Volume 332:170-178

Thomas JL et al (2010). The diagnosis and treatment of heel pain: a clinical practice guideline-revision 2010. Journal of Foot & Ankle Surgery. Volume 49(3 Suppl): S1-S19
van de Water AT, Speksnijder CM. (2010). Efficacy of taping for the treatment of plantar fasciosis: a systematic review of controlled trials. J Am Podiatr Med Assoc. Jan-Feb;100(1):41-51.

Windt et al. (1999) Ultrasound therapy for musculoskeletal disorders: a systematic review. *Pain.*

Zhang SP., Yip TP., Li QS. (2011). Acupuncture treatment for plantar fasciitis: a randomized controlled trial with six months follow-up. Evid Based Complement Alternat Med: 154108

Printed in Great Britain
by Amazon